Digital Health

Digital Health

Understanding the Benefit-Risk
Patient-Provider Framework

Eric D. Perakslis and Martin Stanley

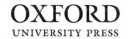

OXFORD
UNIVERSITY PRESS

OXFORD
UNIVERSITY PRESS

Oxford University Press is a department of the University of Oxford. It furthers
the University's objective of excellence in research, scholarship, and education
by publishing worldwide. Oxford is a registered trade mark of Oxford University
Press in the UK and certain other countries.

Published in the United States of America by Oxford University Press
198 Madison Avenue, New York, NY 10016, United States of America.

Library of Congress Cataloging-in-Publication Data
Names: Perakslis, Eric D., author. | Stanley, Martin, 1969– author.
Title: Digital health : understanding the benefit-risk patient-provider
framework / Eric D. Perakslis and Martin Stanley.
Description: New York, NY : Oxford University Press, [2021] |
Includes bibliographical references and index.
Identifiers: LCCN 2020043934 (print) | LCCN 2020043935 (ebook) |
ISBN 9780197503133 (hardback) | ISBN 9780197503140 (paperback) |
ISBN 9780197503164 (epub) | ISBN 9780197503171 (online)
Subjects: MESH: Telemedicine—methods | Risk Assessment | Technology
Assessment, Biomedical | Product Surveillance, Postmarketing | Health
Information Management—methods
Classification: LCC R119.95 (print) | LCC R119.95 (ebook) | NLM W 83.1 |
DDC 610.285—dc23
LC record available at https://lccn.loc.gov/2020043934
LC ebook record available at https://lccn.loc.gov/2020043935

DOI: 10.1093/oso/9780197503133.001.0001

This material is not intended to be, and should not be considered, a substitute for medical or other professional
advice. Treatment for the conditions described in this material is highly dependent on the individual
circumstances. And, while this material is designed to offer accurate information with respect to the subject
matter covered and to be current as of the time it was written, research and knowledge about medical and health
issues is constantly evolving and dose schedules for medications are being revised continually, with new side
effects recognized and accounted for regularly. Readers must therefore always check the product information
and clinical procedures with the most up-to-date published product information and data sheets provided by
the manufacturers and the most recent codes of conduct and safety regulation. The publisher and the authors
make no representations or warranties to readers, express or implied, as to the accuracy or completeness of this
material. Without limiting the foregoing, the publisher and the authors make no representations or warranties as
to the accuracy or efficacy of the drug dosages mentioned in the material. The authors and the publisher do not
accept, and expressly disclaim, any responsibility for any liability, loss, or risk that may be claimed or incurred as a
consequence of the use and/or application of any of the contents of this material.

1 3 5 7 9 8 6 4 2

Paperback printed by LSC Communications, United States of America
Hardback printed by Bridgeport National Bindery, Inc., United States of America

Contents

PART 4: DIGITAL HEALTH—HOPE, HYPE, AND RISK MITIGATION IN PRACTICE

PART 5:   THE FUTURE OF DIGITAL HEALTH BENEFIT-RISK
ASSESSMENT AND MANAGEMENT

Foreword

This book is a field guide to a rapidly developing sector touching all of our lives—digital health—and arrives at an apt moment in time. Though the COVID-19 pandemic has hastened the transition to some forms of digital care, such as telehealth, the shift has not gone as smoothly as hoped. While patients in affluent communities have rapidly adopted telehealth tools that connect them virtually with healthcare workers, patients in rural and low-income urban areas have not been granted the same opportunities.

In addition to exacerbating inequality along racial, geographic, and socioeconomic lines, there are other very real risks associated with the rapid development of digital health technologies. Many of those risks revolve around a central issue: At present, the burden for weighing the harms and benefits of these medical innovations lies not with the medical establishment, nor with federal regulatory bodies. Instead, it falls in the hands of patients—you and me.

We are rapidly becoming what experts in the industry have taken to calling the patient-consumer: We increasingly interact with technological gadgets that double as poorly regulated medical devices. As companies ranging from small startups to corporate giants rush to court us with devices that track our steps, monitor our hearts, gauge our blood pressure, track and deliver our medications, and collect and interpret our DNA, you and I are the ones carrying the most responsibility for determining which devices to use and when, as well as whether those devices are a net benefit to our health and wellbeing or whether their risks outweigh their rewards.

The authors of this book are uniquely equipped to explore these thorny ethical and technological questions. Eric Perakslis and Martin Stanley pioneered technology-driven approaches to the regulation of health technologies at the U.S. Food and Drug Administration (FDA), one of the chief agencies charged with monitoring and regulating these tools. Together, Perasklis and Stanley collectively served in leadership roles at virtually all of the fields relevant to this sector and its rapid uptake, from pharmaceutical companies to startups and federal research agencies.

In this book, Perakslis and Stanley take an unflinching approach to examining the perils and promise of virtual care, issues that I have also addressed in my time as a science and healthcare reporter and editor. Having written in depth about everything from virtual care startups to the development of artificial intelligence (AI)-based hospital decision support tools, I view the issue of unequal access as digital health's primary potential for harm. It is a subject that is explored in detail throughout the chapters ahead.

Digital health is also associated, of course, with huge potential gains and benefits, from faster time to diagnoses to regular monitoring of chronic conditions like diabetes that might otherwise go unchecked, aside from an occasional doctor's visit. The field could also improve overall access to care—especially for stigmatized conditions such as mental health disorders—by meeting patients where they are and being available 24/7. Finally, advanced systems built with AI and machine learning could enhance doctors and radiologists by helping to point out signs of illness that might otherwise go unseen, and flag patients at a high risk of dying to hospital staff to ensure they get immediate care.

Yet it is unclear whether this is, in fact, taking place. The problem is particularly troubling when one considers the ways in which telehealth, arguably the most basic of digital health tools, was heralded at the start of the COVID-19 pandemic as a potential "great equalizer"—a tool that would help even the playing field for everyone, regardless of race, gender, geography, or socioeconomic status.

Fundamental obstacles including a lack of high-speed Internet and basic tools including smartphones and computers have prevented many of the neediest from reaping the benefits of this transformation, although ironically, these communities have also bared a disproportionate burden of COVID-19 infections and deaths. Indeed, more than 25 million people, or 13% of the U.S. population, do not presently have access to broadband, the fast and reliable Internet connection required to use most virtual care platforms (https://www.fcc.gov/document/fcc-releases-2018-broadband-deployment-report).

If patients cannot access this most rudimentary component of digital health, how can they be expected to benefit from the ongoing development of more advanced virtual tools, such as wearable heart rate monitors, "smart" blood pressure cuffs, and connected glucose monitors? Moreover, how can digital health—a field whose many promises includes greater and more equitable access to care—hold up its end of the bargain when simple tools that let patients text or video chat with their practitioners have failed to do so?

Perakslis and Stanley pose these questions with adept authority and come away with unique and critical insights. Their writing addresses a key issue inherent in the field: Patient-consumers are not adequately informed about these tools, including when and where they are being used—including, and most troublingly—in their own care. The regulatory bodies charged with evaluating these tools, including the FDA, have not been able to keep up with the unprecedented pace at which new digital health interventions are being developed and deployed. Amid a global pandemic where clinicians, engineers, and data scientists are rushing to use new solutions, the problem is worsening.

In October 2020, the FDA held a meeting on AI where it grappled with some of the fundamental questions these tools will pose, from their potential to exacerbate bias to the tall task of ensuring patients benefit equally from the tools (https://www.statnews.com/2020/10/26/artificial-intelligence-bias-fda-patients/). But the agency has a long way to go before it is regularly and comprehensively assessing these technologies in a way that serves all patients equally.

The risks are not merely to individual patients, but rather to entire health systems. New devices such as smartwatches already threaten to tip the delicate balance of pressure on the healthcare system by flooding patients with data and increasing the frequency with which they contact clinicians and nurses. Broaches to hospital privacy now unfold with the same regularity as holidays. And many of the AI-powered systems charged with predicting which patients are likely to get worse or die are unproven, with little data showing their real impact on patient care.

Anyone who is interested in healthcare—its past, present, and future—should read this book. The chapters ahead present a runway for clinicians, engineers, academics, and patients to craft a future in which the risks and harms of digital health are outweighed by its promise and potential: healthcare that is more equal and just as well as superior.

Erin Brodwin
Health Tech Reporter and Author
December 2020

Preface

Our Working "Definition" of Digital Health

If you ask "Dr. Google" for a definition of digital health, you will receive numerous and varying answers because there is no universally accepted definition. Some definitions are based upon toolsets. The U.S. Food and Drug Administration (FDA) states that the broad scope of digital health includes, "categories such as mobile health (mHealth), health information technology (IT), wearable devices, telehealth and telemedicine, and personalized medicine."[1] Some definitions are based upon ambition or vison for societal impact, such as that from Mesko and colleagues, "the cultural transformation of how disruptive technologies that provide digital and objective data accessible to both caregivers and patients leads to an equal level doctor-patient relationship with shared decision-making and the democratization of care."[2] Some definitions combine the two, as in, "digital health is the convergence of digital technologies health, healthcare, living, and society to enhance the efficiency of healthcare delivery."[3] The results are even more diverse when we start to compare definitions for Digital Health and Digital Medicine, because those results blend the concepts of digital technology tools with other rapidly evolving medical tools, such as genomics and multimodal health data.[4]

In an effort to achieve a more precise, and it is hoped universally accepted definition, the Healthcare Information and Management Systems Society (HIMSS) has proposed, "Digital health connects and empowers people and populations to manage health and wellness, augmented by accessible and supportive provider teams working within flexible, integrated, interoperable, and digitally-enabled care environments that strategically leverage digital tools, technologies and services to transform care delivery."[5] To tell the truth, I am unsure if this makes things clearer or less so given the length and vagueness. Interestingly, one of the earliest definitions for digital health may still be the best. Writing in 2000, SR Frank described digital health care as the "Convergence of Health Care and the Internet" and further that "interactive media (the Internet and the World Wide Web) and associated applications used to access those media (portals, browsers, specialized Web-based applications) will result in a substantial, positive, and measurable impact on medical care faster than any previous information technology or communications tool."[6] For us, this definition resonates, because it includes the significant impact that Internet browsing has had on patients, providers, and health care.

Given the lack of consensus and our intentions with this book, we have decided to take a very broad approach to what we consider digital health. Key to our approach are Internet connectivity; tools and models that have changed and impacted wellness, health and care delivery; methods of information access by patients, providers, and caregivers; technologies and tools for decision support, such as artificial intelligence and machine learning; tools and models that have enabled remote and virtualized care, and any and all new or traditional associated benefits, harms, or risks.

It is also important to note that we view much of this as simple progression of traditional health care and information tools and technologies. There is no magic here, no unicorns or mythical creatures, although much of the hyperbole is based upon the assumption that a pot of gold lies at the end of the digital health rainbow. For us, these are simply evolved and emerging technology capabilities with great promise, and they should be evaluated, valued, and de-risked using solid and preexisting evaluation frameworks wherever and whenever possible.

References

1. U.S. FDA. Digital Health. Accessed July 2020. https://www.fda.gov/medical-devices/digital-health
2. Meskó B, Z Drobni, É Bényei, B Gergely, and Z Győrffy. 2017. Digital Health Is a Cultural Transformation of Traditional Healthcare. *Mhealth* 2017. 3:38. doi:10.21037/mhealth.2017.08.07.
3. Wikipedia. Digital Health. Accessed July 2020. https://en.wikipedia.org/wiki/Digital_health
4. Topol EJ. A Decade of Digital Medicine Innovation. *Science Translational Medicine* 2019. 11(498):eaaw7610. doi:10.1126/scitranslmed.aaw7610.
5. Cmstock J. HIMSS Launches New Definition of Digital Health. *Mobile Health News.* 2020, March 10.
6. Frank SR. Digital Health Care—The Convergence of Health Care and the Internet. *Journal of Ambulatory Care Management* 2000. 23(2):8–17. doi:10.1097/00004479-200004000-00003

PART 1

HISTORICAL OVERVIEW AND THE EVOLUTION OF DIGITAL HEALTH TECHNOLOGIES

1

A Brief History of Biomedical Products Regulation

Thoughtful and thorough consideration of digital health requires that the benefits and harms are considered with equal levels of scrutiny. It is very easy to get caught up in the excitement of new healthcare tools and trends. We have all lost people to disease, and we all know many others who are fighting daily battles with illness and injury, including ourselves. The Internet has changed medicine by putting health information at our fingertips at scales that are previously unimaginable The promise of digital technologies can be a siren song, but those of us who have spent our careers in healthcare technology understand that there is a delicate balance. Just as most medicines have accompanying undesirable side effects, so do digital health technologies. The challenge is that we do not fully understand them yet. In this chapter, we will start the conversation with a brief review of biomedical products regulation as a first step toward managing the benefits and risks of digital health solutions.

Overview of medical safety

The World Health Organization (WHO) estimates that approximately 43 million medical adverse events occur annually out of 421 million hospitalizations worldwide. This 1-out-of-10 harm rate makes patient harm the 14th greatest disease burden worldwide.[1] Economically, this consumes roughly 15% of healthcare spending overall. Among the most common adverse events are hospital infections at 14 out of every 100 hospitalizations, more than 1 million deaths per year due to surgical complications, and significant rates of misdiagnosis and administrative error. As impressive and scary as these numbers are, the truth is that they are considered low estimates due to significant underreporting.

In the United States, the numbers are equally sobering. Estimates from 1997 depict a range between 44,000 and 98,000 Americans dying annually as a result of medical errors.[2] One study in 2016 by a team from Johns Hopkins

Digital Health. Eric D. Perakslis and Martin Stanley, Oxford University Press (2021). © Oxford University Press.
DOI: 10.1093/oso/9780197503133.003.0001

claimed that the rates were much higher and that medical errors may be the third highest cause of death.[3] The team reasoned that the methods employed by the Centers for Disease Control and Prevention (CDC) underestimate, because medical errors are not classified separately on death certificates. Despite this significant error rate, 90% of deaths are not caused by medical error or adverse events and as such should not be reason to avoid healthcare interventions. So how are the risks and benefits of medical intervention calculated? The answer is complicated, given that the earliest practices of medicine focused on unmet medical need with far less thought for the potential harms.

A brief history of medical products regulation

For most of human history, there was no concept of, or formalized code for, consumer protection. Ancient notions of *caveat emptor*, let the buyer beware, are taught in primary school today and were based upon the fact that a seller usually knows more about a given product than a buyer. Interestingly, the first instance of caveat emptor executed into written law in 1603 involved the sale of a stone that forms in the intestinal track of animals and was believed to have healing properties.[4] In this case, the stone was found not to have magical properties or to even be the type of stone claimed, but the judgment was for the seller because it was ruled the burden of proof was placed upon the buyer. In the United States, this approach prevailed until the first consumer protection agency, the Federal Trade Commission (FTC) was created on September 26, 1914 by President Woodrow Wilson with the mission to protect consumers and promote competition.[5] With respect to medical products, the U.S. Food and Drug Administration (FDA) formally emerged out of the Department of Agriculture (DoA) in 1930, although many of its current functions originated in the DoA with the passage of the Pure Food and Drugs Act in 1906.[6]

The basics of early drug regulation centered upon ensuring medicines were properly labeled and conformed to the applicable standard compendia. There were no requirements for safety, efficacy, or usefulness. Despite early regulatory efforts, these gaps remained unchanged until 1937, when a manufacturer introduced an untested formulation of sulfanilamide with a solvent that was responsible for the deaths of over 100 people.[7] This event prompted President Roosevelt to sign the Food, Drug and Cosmetic Act, which revamped the oversight of food and drugs and began oversight of cosmetics and medical devices for the first time. Most importantly, this law established the requirements and practices of mandatory premarket review to prove the safety of a new drug before it could be placed on the market. The next major event was the inclusion of drug efficacy into the regulations in 1962 to show the drug provided benefit. This major change was born of a Congressional investigation launched by Senator Estes Kefauver in the late 1950s into the effectiveness of drugs and was the birth of modern clinical trials.[8] Concurrently, the linkage of birth defects to the drug thalidomide, which affected more than 10,000 children, was made in 1961, after the drug had been in use for years.[9]

Despite efforts to police medical "devices" such as nose straighteners, height-stretching machines, and devices emitting dangerous radiation that carried claims of prevention of appendicitis and/or gallbladder disease, dating back to the 1930s, medical-device-regulation authority did not arrive at the FDA until 1976. The authority to review and approve radiation-emitting devices arrived via the Radiation Control for Health and Safety Act of 1968, and the authority to regulate medical devices came later via the 1976 Medical Device Amendments.[10] As we move on to study modern digital health, these histories are extremely important. First, although claims made about fraudulent devices of 100 years ago may seem silly today, many consumers have no idea how modern digital devices work or of the associated hazards. Second, the important differences of FDA policing versus regulating are key, because new product types are usually policed before they are regulated. Policing, as the FDA did early on with medical devices, is retrospective. The FDA must observe and study harms prior to prosecution, but this starts *after* the product is on the market. A modern example would be *e*-cigarettes and the issues associated with vaping by minors. None of this was regulated or illegal at the time of product launch, because these items were not explicitly listed within any regulatory statute. Implications of the lack of policing prior to regulation is that harms must occur before action can be taken.

Consumer protection versus health care

Another interesting and important aspect of biomedical-product regulation in the United States is the unobvious dichotomy in the mission of the FDA. Is the FDA a healthcare agency, responsible for improving the health of Americans, or is it a consumer protection agency, responsible for regulating biomedical products but without an opinion on healthcare policy? These are far from being the same thing. For example, in the case of new immunotherapies for cancer, is it the job of the FDA to review each one in isolation and assess only if each is safe or effective, which would be consumer protection, or is it also the job of the FDA to determine which one is best and for which patient, which would be health care? The short answer is that comparative effectiveness, in general, is not part of the FDA's mission, although there are exceptions for certain types of regulatory filings. The underlying issues for this conflict of purpose are complex and have their basis in sociology and in statute.

The FDA is an agency within the U.S. Department of Health and Human Services (HHS) that is presided over by the Secretary of HHS, a presidential appointee. This makes the FDA, and the other healthcare agencies of HHS, subject to the political agenda of any sitting president. Practically speaking, most of the activities of these and other federal agencies, and their employees, are protected from political influence by legislation such as the Hatch Act.[11] However, health is one of the most controversial and politicized aspects of our society, and political influence is an accepted aspect of health regulation. This becomes relevant and important in several key ways. First, even excellent and objective scientific assessment of safety and efficacy can run afoul of public sentiment. Second, as has been notable with the saga of hydroxychloroquine during the COVID-19 pandemic, the agency must walk a fine line between political allegiance and scientific integrity.[12] We will discuss this dichotomy in more detail and specificity as we proceed through specific medical product types.

References

1. World Health Organization. 10 Facts on Patient Safety. September 2019. https://www.who. int/features/factfiles/patient_safety/en/
2. National Academies of Medicine. To Err is Human: Building a Safer Health System. 1999. http://www.nationalacademies.org/hmd/Reports/1999/To-Err-is-Human-Building-A-Safer-Health-System.aspx
3. Makary M. Study Suggests Medical Errors Now Third Leading Cause of Death in the U.S. *Johns Hopkins Medicine*, May 2016.
4. *Chandelor v Lopus*. Wikipedia. Accessed September 2019. https://en.wikipedia.org/wiki/Chandelor_v_Lopus
5. Federal Trade Commission. Our History. December 2017. https://www.ftc.gov/about-ftc/our-history
6. U.S. FDA. The History of FDA's Fight for Consumer Protection. June 2018. https://www.fda. gov/about-fda/history-fdas-fight-consumer-protection-and-public-health
7. U.S. FDA. NDA Approvals and Receipts since 1938. January 2018. https://www.fda.gov/about-fda/histories-product-regulation/summary-nda-approvals-receipts-1938-present
8. White-Junod S. FDA and Clinical Drug Trials: A Short History. Accessed October 2019. https://www.fda.gov/media/110437/download
9. Science Museum. (n.d.). Science Museum. Brought to Life: Exploring the History of Medicine. Accessed November 20, 2019. http://broughttolife.sciencemuseum.org.uk/broughttolife/themes/controversies/thalidomide

10. U.S.FDA.MedicalDevice&RadiologicalHealthRegulationsComeofAge.January2018.https:// www.fda.gov/about-fda/histories-product-regulation/medical-device-radiological- health-regulations-come-age
11. U.S. FDA. The Hatch Act: Political Activity and the Federal Employee. September 2019. https://www.fda.gov/about-fda/ethics/hatch-act-political-activity-and-federal-employee
12. Herper M. A Flawed COVID-19 Study Gets the White House's Attention—and the FDA May Pay the Price. *STAT News*. 2020, July 8.

2

Medical Benefit-Risk Determination

Benefit-risk determination for medical products is a highly complex mix of art and science, in which risks tend to be far more difficult to quantify than benefits and often are revealed years after product approval. Further, side effects often occur in systems other than the system of action of a product. A classic example of drug side effects is heart arrhythmia caused by arthritis medicine. During research and development, the drug likely was studied extensively in the skeletal and immunological systems but not necessarily in the circulatory system. We are at a similar stage of learning with digital health. We all have reaped the benefits of "Dr Google," but we also have seen the rise of truly harmful medical misinformation. We have come to enjoy social media as a positive part of our lives, but we read daily stories of these companies selling our personal information without our permission. In this chapter, we will review the basics of medical product benefit risk with an eye toward the development of understanding the risks and potential harms of digital health technologies.

The opportunity and challenge of benefit-risk determination

For nonmedical professionals, it is easy to imagine that medical benefit risk is something readily quantified and consistently managed. Nothing could be further from the truth. Medical care is dynamic and uncertain. Regardless of the number of patients studied in clinical trials and even after decades of use, any given patient may react differently, favorably or unfavorably, to any given treatment, and medical professionals must assess and act on the fly. Hence, in practice, medical benefit risk is subjective and, often, anecdotal. When new treatments or new combinations or varieties of existing treatments are first launched, they are introduced with great caution. Every healthcare practitioner must decide when, where, and how to utilize new tools, often with just basic, and potentially biased by marketing, guidance. Patients themselves are often, and appropriately, brought into the conversation, "the older drug often causes this side effect. The newer drug claims not to, but I haven't tried it yet

Digital Health. Eric D. Perakslis and Martin Stanley, Oxford University Press (2021). © Oxford University Press.
DOI: 10.1093/oso/9780197503133.003.0002

in any of my patients. What do you think?" Clearly, benefit-risk determination involves all stakeholders in the healthcare process but creating and mobilizing this diverse community in a productive way requires the collection and sharing of a large amount and variety of data.

Each of these stakeholder groups is increasing its demands for data to support decision-making, and more and more types of real-world data are available every day. Examples of data being electronically collected and tracked include electronic health record (EHR) data, Medicare claims data, patient-reported outcomes, clinical trials data, Food and Drug Administration (FDA) medical safety surveillance data, patient and clinician-run disease registries, genetics and molecular profiling data, and digital sensor data collected for wellness and health care. As regulators and payers ramp up their calls for better and more quantified benefit-risk information, all of these data can be helpful, but they also pose logistical and technical challenges to product developers that are expected to monitor the health benefits and risks over the entire lifecycle of a product. This is especially challenging given the diversity of benefits and risks in health care. According to Juhn and colleagues,

> Although the benefits related to stopping or slowing disease progression or preventing disease in a patient might be obvious and relatively easy to quantify, the benefits related to the quality of life of the patient or even the caregiver are more subjective, although no less important. The potential for some commonly occurring side effects might be relatively easy to quantify in clinical trials, but many other risks emerge only in real-world experience. Sometimes unique features influence the severity of the risk, such as those associated with the skill of the provider or the number of procedures performed in a particular hospital setting. And sometimes the risks associated with not treating are greater than those associated with a treatment.[1]

This is very well said.

Many are hopeful that digital health will improve medical practice and patient value across the board via improved benefit-risk data and real-time information for clinicians, caregivers, and patients. Indeed, digital tools could be the solution for the inherent data and knowledge management gaps that arise from the need for product developers, clinicians, regulators, payers, and patients to study medical benefit-risk in real time throughout product lifecycle. The rapid appearance of digital health technologies makes proactive study and monitoring essential. Programs such as the Digital Medicine Payment Advisory Group, a collaborative initiative, convened by the American Medical Association (AMA), to study digital health with the goal of creating a clear pathway for the integration of digital medicine technologies into clinical practice are a great example of positive, thoughtful, and proactive action to enable and exploit digital health solutions properly.[2]

In this chapter, we have selected a subset of medical benefit-risk domains to examine. It is not meant to be exhaustive but illustrative of the most common types of benefit-risk determination as well as the variety of domains and situations that could be considered. It is an intentional mix of the traditional and the new with an eye toward the future of patient care.

Drug toxicity and side effects

Despite approximately three and a half years of drug toxicity testing during premarket clinical trials, most adverse drug reactions are not identified until after the drug is marketed.[3,4] There are several reasons for this. First, regulatory approval requires precise studies that clearly demonstrate the effects, good and bad, of the drug being tested. This leads to a tension between finding a large enough group of patients to demonstrate these effects without including populations that could confound the analysis. Specifically, during the design of a trial, researchers must select for patients who clearly have the condition they intend to treat, they must represent the specific subsegment of that patient population, they cannot have complex or confounding comorbidities, and cannot be on other medications that could mask or confound the effect of the drug being tested, as well as many other complex criteria.[5] This leads to trial designs that can appear to have impossibly narrow patient enrollment criteria. Unavoidable challenges in premarket safety testing include the poor translatability of cellular and animal studies to humans and the limited time frames of clinical trials.[6] Early toxicology studies are designed to identify major safety issues. Timing of the developmental toxicology studies is determined by the inclusion of women of childbearing potential (WCBP) in early clinical trials. Depending on the target indication, this may not happen until after the drug is marketed. The acceptable duration of nonrodent chronic toxicology studies is nine months to one year. Depending on the therapeutic indication, carcinogenicity studies may be conducted after approval (Phase IV), if there is no special cause for concern in that regard.

Food and Drug Administration labeling and postmarketing surveillance

One of the penultimate outcomes of the FDA drug approval process is an approved label. The prescription drug labels are highly regulated and include

Prescribing Information (PI); FDA-approved patient labeling (Medication Guides, Instructions for Use, and Patient Information [also called Patient Package Inserts]); carton and container labeling; and promotional materials accompanying the product.[7] Labels are living documents because, especially for newer drugs, they are almost always in a state of change as experience with the product evolves. Examples of the changes include modifications in dosing, safety information and side effects, and expansion of access to new populations. Once the drug and label are fully approved, safety surveillance switches to what is called postmarket surveillance.

After a newly approved drug enters the marketplace, postmarketing experience can reveal adverse events (AEs) not detected during clinical trials or preapproval review. The FDA maintains two major systems for postmarketing drug surveillance, a "passive" system known as FAERS (FDA Adverse Event Reporting System) and an "active" system known as the Sentinel System.[8] It is important to understand that this process is a mix of mandatory reporting from sponsors and voluntary reporting from anyone, although most of the voluntary reports are discharged and eventually not loaded into the database, due to incompleteness, inaccuracy, or events that already have been proven to be untrue. The FDA does keep data on the most recent safety elements of medical products readily available to patients and healthcare providers on a dedicated webpage.[9]

Safety event reporting has very specific requirements based upon the severity of AEs. Critical to note is that the time requirements for reporting become shorter as the seriousness of the AE increases.[10] The principles behind processes are typical for safety surveillance of biomedical products and benefit-risk determination: (i) manufacturers retain perpetual responsibility for the safety and use of their products; (ii) the severity of a safety incident determines timeline and extent of data required in reporting; (iii) voluntary reporting from patients, clinicians, and caregivers follows a separate process but ends up in the same data set if proven to be accurate.

Medical adverse events and errors: introduction and definition

Revisiting medical harm, there are various definitions and contexts to consider. The term medical AE has multiple definitions. The FDA and the Code of Federal Regulations (CFR) define AEs as "any untoward medical occurrence associated with the use of a drug in humans, whether or not considered drug related."[11] This is obviously a drug-centric view, but the definition carries over into the medical device domains where events such as device malfunctions may or may not have caused direct or indirect patient harm.[12] For this reason, many use the term adverse drug event (ADE) when specifically speaking to medication adverse events. The various types of adverse events can be further classified as preventable or nonpreventable, with preventable AEs being described as "avoidable by any means currently available unless that means was not considered standard care."[13] A nonpreventable AE is a drug reaction that occurs in a patient who has been appropriately prescribed a drug for the first time, but one that is unavoidable given what is currently known at the time of the event.[14] Adverse events are commonly referred to as side effects. Preventable AEs are typically defined as care that fell below the standard expected of physicians in their community. Preventable AEs also are often referred to as medical errors and can be errors of commission or omission. Whether preventable or not, medical AEs are a significant source of patient risk and warrant constant study, monitoring, and mitigation.

Adverse drug events are much more common than many would suspect, causing nearly 700,000 emergency room visits and 100,000 hospitalizations per year.[15] This should not be too surprising given an armamentarium of more than 10,000 available medicines and with nearly one-third of adults in the United States taking five or more of these medicines. The probabilities of ADEs rise significantly as patients are prescribed more medications for a single condition, a concept known as polypharmacy, or for multiple conditions.

Measurement, probability, and prevention of adverse events

Two of the most essential elements in the measurement and characterization of medical AEs are time and precision. The more precisely AEs can be described and quantified, the larger the number of variables that are available to manipulate for prevention. For many AEs, the time allowed for measurement and investigation of AEs is codified in regulatory statute by product type. For example, the U.S. FDA lists postmarketing reporting requirements by product type and the specific governing law on its website.[16] As with medical devices, the extent of data required and the required time limit for reporting are based upon the seriousness of the AE. Current ADE definitions/classifications include *life-threatening, serious, suspected,* and *unexpected.* These definitions are obviously subject to interpretation. Looking more closely at serious AEs, the FDA describes them as,

An adverse event or suspected adverse reaction is considered "serious" if, in the view of either the investigator or sponsor, it results in any of the following outcomes: Death, a life-threatening adverse event, inpatient hospitalization or prolongation of existing hospitalization, a persistent or significant incapacity or substantial disruption of the ability to conduct normal life functions, or a congenital anomaly/birth defect. Important medical events that may not result in death, be life-threatening, or require hospitalization may be considered serious when, based upon appropriate medical judgment, they may jeopardize the patient or subject and may require medical or surgical intervention to prevent one of the outcomes listed in this definition.[17]

Medical device reporting requirements (MDR) codes are shown in Table 2.1 to demonstrate the differences between drug and medical device AE reporting.[18]

Frankly, we believe that these two tables should be on full display in every tech startup that seeks to "fix" medicine with novel technology.

Lastly, beyond the regulatory obligations of biomedical product researchers, manufacturers, and importers, healthcare professionals also play an important role in the safety surveillance of medical products. The AMA specifies the responsibility of reporting medical AEs directly within the ethics sections of its webpage.[19] This is an excellent approach and one that should be emulated

Table 2.1 Categories of FDA Medical Device Reporting Codes

Name	Purpose
Device Problem Code	Describe device failure or issues related to the device during the reported event through observational language
Manufacture Evaluation Method Code	Describe the method of investigation of the device involved in the reported event
Manufacture Evaluation Result Code	Describe specific findings from the investigation of the device involved in the reported event, typically an explanation for the device problem observed
Manufacturer Evaluation Conclusion Code	Describe conclusions from the investigation of the device involved in the reported event, typically a root cause for the device problem observed
Patient Problem Code	Describe actual adverse effects on a patient that may be related to the device problem observed during the reported event
Device Component code	Describe specific device components or assemblies associated with the device problem observed during the reported event

across the health ecosystem, including the rapidly evolving digital health eco-system, as we will discuss later.

The only way to reliably prevent medical errors and AEs is to understand causality at the most fundamental levels. There are many causal factors and a great deal of specificity to the causes and effects of errors in medicine. One common approach is to classify errors as active or latent, wherein active failures are the unsafe acts committed by people who are in direct contact with the patient or system. Latent conditions are the inevitable "resident pathogens" within the system.[20,21] By thinking of medical errors as human or structurally based, we can be one step closer to understanding and mitigation. Human errors often are classified as personal or systems based. The personal approach focuses on the errors of individuals, blaming them for forgetfulness, inattention, or moral weakness, while the system approach concentrates on the conditions under which individuals work and tries to build defenses to avert errors or mitigate their effects.[22] The confounder here is that human-based errors often are caused by structural issues, which we argue are more likely when employing emerging technology in new and highly complex domains such as medicine. This important interplay and/or interdependency has been called out in a Stanford Medical study, which determined that physician burnout is at least equally responsible for medical errors as unsafe medical workplace conditions, if not more so.[23]

Disclosure and benefit risk

Despite a clear moral imperative to disclose medical errors and AEs, actual practices appear to vary greatly by institution and subspecialty. The American College of Physicians ethics manual states, "Physicians should disclose to patients information about procedural or judgment errors made during care, as long as such information is material to the patient's well-being. Errors do not necessarily imply negligent or unethical behavior, but failure to disclose them may be."[24] Despite this and similar guidance, the general perception is that most errors go undisclosed to patients. One recent Swiss study to test a set of formalized medical error disclosure competence guidelines (MEDC) found that, although one in four patients had experienced a medical error during the past five years of their medical care, only every third of these patients received a disclosure.[25]

The primary driver for the lack of disclosure appears to be liability/malprac-tice concerns. Indeed, taking the lead from several European countries, the concern that clinician disclosure or apology may be used against a clinician in court is so prevalent that many U.S. states are considering medical professional apology statutes that will ensure disclosures or apology statements themselves cannot be used as evidence in court procedings.[26] To date, approximately 40 states have adopted some form of apology law. That said, in the United Kingdom, the presence of these apology statutes does not appear adequate to assure clinicians protection from the potential legal consequences of disclosure.[27] In one extremely high-profile case in the United Kingdom, a pediatrician trainee was blamed for the death of a six-year-old boy and faced a series of legal and disciplinary processes, which included a conviction for negligent manslaughter and removal from the medical register, despite the reported presence of significant systems failures outside the control of the trainee that contributed to this very sad event.[28] This case highlights the reasons why many physicians may be disinclined to disclose medical errors, as has been the approach for most of modern medical history. In fact, the infamous traditional approach recommended by medical malpractice defense lawyers is known as "deny and defend," clearly the exact opposite of what virtually all medical ethics training and statutes implore.[29]

These concepts are relevant as we consider digital health, wherein a much greater responsibility lies with the patient for proper and appropriate use of tools that are minimally clinician supervised.

Quantitative methods for calculating medical benefit risk

Traditional assessment of medical benefit risk requires detailed and quantitative understandings of the many individual types of medical benefits and medical risks but is often limited to qualitative oversimplifications due to the complexities of the resulting math. The need to simplify the complexities of medical benefit risk into simple metrics that are easily translatable to clinical care can promote assumptions that omit complex concepts and variables in the effort to make the measures accessible to the intended patient populations. This in and of itself is not a bad thing, because these stakeholders' input is necessary to maintain performance measures that can be measured, tracked, and managed. Simple metrics, especially with new and novel treatment and diagnostic modalities, tend to work best but require surveillance themselves in order to validate that they are effective and complete. The assessment of benefit risk in digital health adds layers of new complexity to these calculations because: (i) novel digital health measures and endpoints may have very limited data availability; (ii) the measures themselves may be new and poorly understood; and (iii) the environmental risks of Internet connectivity and dependency present new and difficult-to-predict harms, and the technologies are often new and unproven. An excellent example of a quantitative assessment of benefits and harms has been provided by Snappin and Jiang.[30] In summary, the simplified case defines the benefits and harms each as single absolute time-to-event variables, which depict the number of participants who experience an event and how long it takes for that event to occur. It also is assumed that the variables are statistically independent and that they are of equal importance.

First, it is important to understand the key terms and variables used in benefit-risk determination. Benefit-risk determination often is studied via survival analysis, which is defined as methods for analyzing data where the outcome variable is the time until the occurrence of an event of interest. The event can be death, occurrence of a disease, marriage, divorce, etc. The time to event or survival time can be measured in days, weeks, years, etc.[31] In survival analysis, the hazard ratio (HR) is the ratio of the hazard rates corresponding to the conditions described by two levels of an explanatory variable. For example, in a drug study, the treated population may die at twice the rate per unit time as the control population. An HR of 1 means that both groups (treatment and control) are experiencing an equal number of events at any point in time. An HR of 0.333 tells you that the hazard rate in the treatment group is one third of that in the control group. These calculations are used to estimate the individual risks involved, such as risk of treatment, risk of nontreatment, and additional other effects, and the final determination is about a combination of these individual risk differences.

The challenges of quantifying risks and harms

From a global health perspective, studies have identified childhood and maternal underweight, unsafe sex, high blood pressure, tobacco, and alcohol as the leading causes of burdens of disease.[32] Further, as previously cited, the World Health Organization (WHO) lists patient harm as the fourteenth leading cause of global disease burden with confirmed incidence of AEs occurring in one out of ten hospitalizations.[33] It also must be assumed that the actual numbers are likely higher, given that most accidents in hospitals are believed to go unreported, and that AEs in clinical trials may be underreported by at least 83% in unpublished clinical studies.[34,35] Estimates of medical harms from outside of the clinic are even more difficult to assess. For patients with serious illnesses being treated at home via professional homecare services, one

Swedish study found an AE rate of 37.7% with 71.6% of these being assessed as preventable.[36]

With respect to unsupervised medical care at home, as in the case of many digital health applications, estimates are far less straightforward. First, patient "user error" and compliance are difficult to quantify. Second, the fact that many patients are being seen by a variety of specialists increases the probability of unanticipated polypharmacy risks, risks associated with drug-drug interactions.[37] Third, existing reporting systems are not suited to capture the complex nature of ADEs or adapted to workflow and are simply not used by frontline clinicians.[38] Fourth, and possibly most importantly, it is nobody's job to report medical AEs outside of supervised medical care. Most recently, the backstop for this gap has been retrospective study of electronic health records, especially in primary care, but this remains a nascent practice at best. One Dutch study reported a two-fold difference in general practices in measuring medication-based AEs.[39] So, without the oversight of clearly responsible parties or readily available systems, it is very difficult to assess medical safety in the course of daily life at home.

Further, as shown in the examples above, if medical risk is typically determined as difference in probabilities between compared groups of patients, such as control groups, placebo groups, etc., it is infeasible to apply these same approximations to daily-life settings. Lastly, in assessing the total risk of healthcare accidents and mistakes, at least one group of professionals is keeping score, at least in the United States, and that is medical malpractice attorneys. Often, these groups can be the first point of contact, due to intense solicitation, of patients who feel they have been harmed by medicine.[40] The cases that merit investigation and litigation often are left to the legal system and typically to opposing outside medical expertise to adjudicate. This is clearly a failure of our medical safety net in that the ripple effects of cases inspire defensive medicine that can lead to overdiagnosis and overtreatment, as well as to fear and insecurity that are likely unhelpful with respect to the transparency of medical practice overall.

Risk-management frameworks

Beyond the benefit-risk assessment of a drug modeled in physiological isolation within a single patient, as is the norm in randomized clinical trials where concurrent medications that could lead to drug-drug interactions are often eliminated via patient selection criteria, the risks of any intervention must be considered holistically as patients do not live the idealized environments required for randomized controlled trials (RCTs). This is best accomplished by a comprehensive risk-management plan or framework such as is required by the European Medicines Agency (EMA). For example, the risk management plan (RMP) specified within the EMA good pharmacovigilance practices (GVP) module 5 states that an RMP must contain:

- the identification or characterization of the safety profile of the medicinal product, with emphasis on important identified and important potential risks and missing information, and also on which safety concerns need to be managed proactively or further studied (the "safety specification");
- the planning of pharmacovigilance activities to characterize and quantify clinically relevant risks and to identify new adverse reactions (the "pharmacovigilance plan");
- the planning and implementation of risk minimization measures, including the evaluation of the effectiveness of these activities (the "risk minimization plan").[41]

The approach and practice in the United States are somewhat different because general drug benefit-risk (BR) assessment is handled via the regulatory approval process with any resulting specific risk management information being covered via the FDA label approval process. There are times, however, when the BR profile requires additional caution, most typically when a drug is intended for very serious disease and the drug carries risk of significant side effects. Under these circumstances, the FDA can require a formal Risk Evaluation and Mitigation Strategy (REMS). REMS are based around one or more specific risk mitigation goal(s) and comprise information communicated to and/or required activities to be undertaken by one or more participants (e.g., healthcare providers, pharmacists, patients) who prescribe, dispense, or take the medication. Together, the goal, communications, and/or activities make up the safety strategy.

One of the most complex and confusing incarnations of benefit-risk assessment is value. As a concept, value is difficult to assess outside of health care as traditional views are highly subjective and based upon financial means and personal context. For example, some would look at a certain luxury car as a great value while others would view any car above a certain price point as a luxury. In health care, value is even more complex. First, there are the various stakeholder perspectives to consider. What looks like a good value to a payer may look like inadequate treatment to a clinician. Some, the authors included, believe that the patient perspective is most important given that more that one in four Americans report facing challenges paying for their medical bills and almost 80% of cancer patients report moderate to catastrophic financial burden related to their care. As is typical, the pressure is felt most acutely by the poorest; low-income families often spend more than 20% of their after-tax income on out-of-pocket healthcare spending, even when enrolled in low- or no-deductible plans, often the only plans they can afford.[42] Interestingly, unlike purely physical benefit risk where benefits are easy to calculate and risks are more difficult, with financial benefit and risk, the financial risks are easier to calculate.

Healthcare value frameworks

Estimating the value of healthcare interventions and services is complex on many levels. Due to widely varied religious beliefs, rapidly growing wealth disparity, complex socioeconomic scenarios, political polarization, rampant misinformation, and complex empiricism and mathematics, there are currently no accepted or mature healthcare value frameworks in use today, but there are a large number of starts. A study by Dubois and Westrich, in 2017, studied a series of healthcare value frameworks that are under development using an established set of guiding standards and found that although most of the studied frameworks were not fully mature, some were already operating *de facto* and are influencing healthcare decision-making.[43] They concluded that the many nascent frameworks could be improved by ensuring that assessments of value are separate from assessments of budget impact and affordability, that value assessments should always involve what is most important to patients even when the end user of the framework is a payer, and that value assessments should utilize broad system perspectives in what they assess and how they assess it. Value assessments also should incorporate the understanding that value is dynamic, it should ensure transparency and reproducibility, utilize a diversity of approaches, and acknowledge the need for insurance reform. Indeed, in looking at many of the currently proposed frameworks, it is clear that they are really "frameworks for frameworks" as opposed to actual solutions and that there is much work to do.

Approved with Research and Only in Research approvals

An interesting facet of the National Institute for Health and care Excellence (NICE) in the United Kingdom approach is a set of additional marketing authorization categories that enable a more analog approach to health technology regulation than the more traditional U.S. FDA approach that something is either safe and effective or it is not. In particular, Only in Research (OIR) is defined as a recommendation which states in the guidance section that the technology should not be used routinely unless it is in the context of further research. Approved with Research (AWR) is defined as a recommendation which states in the guidance section that the technology should be used routinely and which recommends further research is conducted. One example of an AWR recommendation in final guidance comes from TA11391 on the use of inhaled insulin. The guidance section recommends the use of inhaled insulin for a specific subgroup of patients and also includes the statement that "Data on the use of inhaled insulin according to this guidance should be collected as part of a coordinated prospective observational study."[44] An example of an OIR guidance is one provided on hearing aids, which stated that "There is insufficient robust scientific evidence to support the nationwide introduction of digital hearing aids at present. Evidence regarding the benefits of digital devices as compared with the current NHS range and to more sophisticated analogue devices, is expected to be available after the completion of research projects currently being undertaken in the UK."[45]

To the authors, these models are fascinating and should be viewed as opportunities to improve the regulatory frameworks for digital health technologies in the United States. Lastly, we also must be honest with ourselves that value assessment and indeed even medicines that have been understood and utilized effectively for decades, such as insulin, are becoming too expensive for many who need them. This demonstrates that the association between need and cost can be perverse based upon market dynamics and profiteering.

References

1. Juhn P., A. Phillips, and K. Buto. Balancing Modern Benefits and Risks. All Stakeholders Bear the Responsibility for Improving the Understanding of Risk-Benefit Information. *Health Affairs* 2007. 26(3):647–652.
2. AMA. Digital Medicine Payment Advisory Group. Accessed October 2019. https://www.ama-assn.org/practice-management/digital/digital-medicine-payment-advisory-group
3. MedicineNet. Drug Approvals from Invention to Market: A 12-Year Trip. Accessed October 2019. https://www.medicinenet.com/script/main/art.asp?articlekey=9877
4. Liu R et al. Data-Driven Prediction of Adverse Drug Reactions Induced by Drug-Drug Interactions. *BMC Pharmacology and Toxicology* 2017. 18:44.
5. Fogel D. Factors Associated with Clinical Trials that Fail and Opportunities for Improving the Likelihood of Success: A Review. *Contemporary Clinical Trials Communication* 2018. September 11:156–164.

6. Dorato M, and L Buckley. Toxicology Testing in Drug Discovery and Development. *Current Protocols in Toxicology* 2007. February; Chapter 19: Unit19.1.

7. U.S. FDA. Prescription Drug Labeling Resources. Accessed August 2019. https://www.fda.gov/drugs/laws-acts-and-rules/prescription-drug-labeling-resources

8. U.S. FDA CDER. 2015–2016 Drug Safety Priorities Initiatives and Innovation. Accessed September 2019. https://www.fda.gov/media/100679/download

9. U.S. FDA. Postmarket Safety Information for Patients and Providers. Accessed October 2019. https://www.fda.gov/drugs/drug-safety-and-availability/postmarket-drug-safety-information-patients-and-providers

10. U.S. FDA. Mandatory Reporting Requirements: Manufacturers, Importers and Device User Facilities. Accessed October 2019. https://www.fda.gov/medical-devices/postmarket-requirements-devices/mandatory-reporting-requirements-manufacturers-importers-and-device-user-facilities

11. U.S. FDA. CFR–Code of Federal Regulations. [Title 21, Volume 5] [Revised as of April 1, 2019] [CITE: 21CFR312.32].

12. U.S. FDA. CFR–Code of Federal Regulations. [Title 21, Volume 8] [Revised as of April 1, 2019] [CITE: 21CFR803.3].

13. AHRQ. Adverse Events, Near Misses and Errors. Accessed September 2019. https://psnet.ahrq.gov/primers/primer/34/Adverse-Events-Near-Misses-and-Errors

14. Brennan T et al. Incidence of Adverse Events and Negligence in Hospitalized Patients—Results of the Harvard Medical Practice Study I. *New England Journal of Medicine* 1991. 324:370–376.

15. AHRQ. Medication Errors and Adverse Drug Events. Accessed September 2019. https://psnet.ahrq.gov/primers/primer/23/Medication-Errors-and-Adverse-Drug-Events

16. U.S. FDA. Postmarket Drug Safety Information for Patients and Providers. Accessed September 2019. https://www.fda.gov/drugs/drug-safety-and-availability/postmarket-drug-safety-information-patients-and-providers

17. U.S. FDA. CFR–Code of Federal Regulations. [Title 21, Volume 5] [Revised as of April 1, 2019] [CITE: 21CFR312.32]

18. U.S. FDA. MDR Adverse Event Codes. 2018 March. https://www.fda.gov/medical-devices/mandatory-reporting-requirements-manufacturers-importers-and-device-user-facilities/mdr-adverse-event-codes

19. AMA. Required Reporting of Adverse Events. Code of Medical Ethics Opinion 8.8. Accessed October 2019. https://www.ama-assn.org/delivering-care/ethics/required-reporting-adverse-events

20. Pietra LL et al. Medical Errors and Clinical Risk Management: State of the Art. *Acta Otorhinolaryngologica Italica* 2005. 25:339–346.

21. Chang A, PM Schyve, RJ Croteau, DS O'Leary, and JM Loeb. The JCAHO Patient Safety Event Taxonomy: A Standardized Terminology and Classification Schema for Near Misses and Adverse Events. *International Journal for Quality in Health Care* 2005. 17:95–105.

22. Reason J. Human Error: Models and Management. *BMJ* 2000. 320(7237):768–70. doi:10.1136/bmj.320.7237.768

23. Tawfik DS et al. Physician Burnout, Well-being, and Work Unit Safety Grades in Relationship to Reported Medical Errors. *Mayo Clinic Proceedings* 2018. 93(11):1571–1580.

24. American College of Physicians. *American College of Physicians Ethics Manual*, 4th ed. *Annals of Internal Medicine* 1998. 128:576–594.

25. Hannawa A. When Facing Our Fallibility Constitutes "Safe Practice": Further Evidence for the Medical Error Disclosure Competence (MEDC) Guidelines. *Patient Education and Counseling*. 2019. 102(10):1840–1846.

26. National Conference of State Legislators. Medical Professional Apologies Statutes. Accessed October 2019. http://www.ncsl.org/research/financial-services-and-commerce/medical-professional-apologies-statutes.aspx

27. Leung GKK. Safety of Candor: How Protected Are Apologies in Open Disclosure? *BMJ* 2019. 365:l4047.

28. Campbell D. Where Does the Blame Lie When Something Goes Wrong at Hospital? *The Guardian*. 2018, August 13.

29. Boothman RC. CANDOR: The Antidote to Deny and Defend? *Health Services Research* 2016. 51:2487–2490.

30. Snappin S and Q. Jiang. *Benefit-Risk Assessment Methods in Medical Product Development. Bridging Qualitative and Quantitative Assessments*. (Chapman & Hall/CRC Biostatistics Series). Boca Raton, FL. 2016.

31. Altman DJ and JM Bland. Time to Event Survival Data. *BMJ* 1998. 317:468.

32. Ezzati M et al. Selected Major Risk Factors and Global and Regional Burden of Disease. Lancet. 2002. 360(9343):1347–1360.

33. World Health Organization. 10 Facts on Patient Safety. Accessed September 2019. https://www.who.int/features/factfiles/patient_safety/en/

34. U.S. HHS Office of the Inspector General. Hospital Incident Reporting Systems Do Not Capture Most Patient Harms. Accessed August 2019. https://oig.hhs.gov/oei/reports/oei-06-09-00091.asp

35. Golder S et al. Reporting of Adverse Events in Published and Unpublished Studies of Health Care Interventions: A Systematic Review. *PloS Medicine* 2016. 13(9):e1002127.

36. Schildmeijer KGI, M. Unbeck, M. Ekstedt, M. Lindblad, and L. Nilsson. Adverse Events in Patients in Home Healthcare: A Retrospective Record Review Using Trigger Tool Methodology. *BMJ Open* 2018. 8(1):e019267.

37. Dagli RJ and A Sharma. Polypharmacy: A Global Risk Factor for Elderly People. *Journal of International Oral Health* 2014. 6(6):i–ii.

38. Hohl CM, SS Small, D Peddie, K Badke, C Bailey, and E Balka. Why Clinicians Don't Report Adverse Drug Events: Qualitative Study. *JMIR Public Health Surveillance* 2018. 4(1):e21.

39. deHoon SEM, K Hek, L van Dijk, and RA Verhejj. Adverse Events Recording in Electronic Health Record Systems in Primary Care. *BMC Medical Informatics and Decision Making* 2017. 17(1):163.

40. Gilreath and Associates. 8 Common Medical Errors That Can Destroy Lives. Accessed August 2019. https://www.sidgilreath.com/learn/common-medical-errors.html

41. European Medicines Agency. Guidance on the Format of the Risk Management Plan (RMP) in the EU–In Integrated Format. 31 October 2018. EMA/164014/2018 Rev.2.0.1 accompanying GVP Module V Rev.2 Human Medicines Evaluation.

42. Siedman J et al. Measuring Value Based On What Matters To Patients: A New Value Assessment Framework. *Health Affairs Blog*, May 2017.

43. Dubois RW and K Westrich. Value Assessment Frameworks: How Can They Meet The Challenge? *Health Affairs Blog*, March 2017.

44. NICE. Inhaled Insulin for the Treatment of Type 1 and Type 2 Diabetes. TA113. London: NICE; 2006.

45. NICE. Hearing Disability–Hearing Aids (withdrawn). TA8. London: NICE; 2000.

3

Medical Ethics Models and Frameworks in Digital Health

Although neither author is an academically trained ethicist, we are both highly experienced technologists and have spent decades wrestling with the ethical elements of our profession. This chapter will quickly review the core principles of medical ethics but will mostly serve as a basis for a practitioners' guide and playbook to the complex and rapidly evolving ethical issues of digital health.

Backstory: When technological experimentation is human subjects research

In my early days of hospital engineering, I spent almost a year implementing the first carbon dioxide (CO_2) surgical lasers in an operating room of a large community hospital. In the mid-1980s, CO_2 lasers were becoming well understood and usage was expanding quickly. According to VC Wright, writing in the *Journal of the Canadian Medical Association* in 1982, "The CO_2 laser beam is directed through the viewing system of an operating microscope or through a hand-held laser component. Its basic action in tissue is thermal vaporization; it causes minimal damage to adjacent tissues. Surgeons require special training in the basic methods and techniques of laser surgery, as well as in the safety standards that must be observed."[1] The implementation was highly targeted toward vocal cord polyps surgery, which is still a common application today.

A severe risk of this application was endotracheal (ET) tube fires, a challenge that remains today.[2] The issue is caused by the close proximity of the lesions to be ablated and the plastic tube containing a moist, oxygen-enriched gas, creating the possibility that the laser beam will impact the tube causing fire in the airways of the patient. A truly horrible event to imagine. There were no established risk mitigation protocols, so surgeons, anesthesiologists, and biomedical engineers, including us, were experimenting in real time. As an

Digital Health. Eric D. Perakslis and Martin Stanley, Oxford University Press (2021). © Oxford University Press.
DOI: 10.1093/oso/9780197503133.003.0003

engineering undergraduate, I had not yet had any training or exposure to human subjects research or medical ethics and simply did as I was instructed. I still wince about it today . . . .

We actively tested two methodologies to reduce the risk of ET tube fires. First, as the laser beam reflected off of metal, we wrapped ET tubes in metallic foil tape. This approach protected the airway but did carry the risk that the beam could deflect from the tape and cause a burn elsewhere in the surgical field. The second approach was the brainchild of one surgeon in particular who theorized that the risk could be lessened by reducing the oxygen concentration within the ET tube. He tested various methods for accomplishing this, primarily by fabricating a curved metal tube that could be used as a venturi, a method of increasing gas velocity by passing it through a constricted opening. Operationally, this looked a lot like artificial respiration where a puff of gas would be given to the patient, only briefly raising the oxygen concentration in the ET tube, followed by a few seconds of laser work, followed by a puff of oxygen again and the process was repeated throughout the surgical procedure.

Frankly, these processes terrified me. I have vivid memories of sitting for hours with a roll of thin metallic tape in one hand and a plastic ET tube in the other knowing that any gaps in my wrapping could lead to a fire in the throat of a patient. Visualize wrapping a long, curved tube that was approximately eight to ten inches long with a foil tape approximately a quarter inch in width. This process required a lot of wraps, kept neat and sufficiently overlapped with adequate tension, to not slip anywhere causing an opening. It was impossible to do perfectly.

Thankfully, we never did have an ET tube fire during my years at that particular hospital, but the experience has stuck with me for decades and has served as a reference case for my own development and understanding of ethical human subjects research. This is not because I am convinced what we were doing was wrong, but because I simply did not know what risks has been communicated to the patient and which had not. Had the patients fully understood the risks and had they consented? If the patient had consented, did they truly understand what they were agreeing to? Lastly, before passing judgment, it is important to recognize that today's highly evolved practices of ethical medical research were less developed at that time. According to the "History of Informed Consent," published by Peter M. Murray in 1990, there were two interesting court rulings on surgical informed consent around this time, 1985 and 1986, and both limited the burden of risk disclosure of surgeons at the time of surgical consent.[3] The times have changed and, thankfully, so have the practices and obligations of ethical informed consent and risk disclosure. Today things are more evolved but still far from perfect.

One last lesson from this example is that the utilization of technologies can rapidly evolve once they are placed into medical practice. I do not have first-hand knowledge, but I suspect that the lasers we were using were approved by the Food and Drug Administration (FDA) for use in indications and settings such as ours. Interestingly, I also suspect that the ET tube fire was not an issue that was studied during the FDA premarket approval of the laser, because to safely ablate human tissue is not itself overly hazardous. What is hazardous is the application, ablating human tissue next to an oxygen-rich plastic tube inserted into the airway of an anesthetized patient. To this day, approved medical products are frequently marketed for applications that have not been studied for safety and efficacy. For example, on July 30, 2018, the FDA issued a Safety Communication warning against the use of energy-based devices, such as CO_2 lasers, to perform vaginal "rejuvenation" or vaginal cosmetic procedures because the safety and efficacy of these tools is unknown for these applications.[4] I think we must accept that some things may never change, namely, that new medical technologies will be marketed for unstudied or understudied applications and that the FDA always will be playing catch-up.

The four pillars of medical ethics

According to Dr. Paul Niselle, writing for medicalprotection.org, "Medical practice is an ethical and legal minefield. So, what helps us manage these dilemmas in an effective way? The answer is—rarely, the law, but commonly, ethics."[5] This statement is useful because it captures the vital essence of complexity when it comes to ethics and legality—it's complicated.

Starting with the basics of medical ethics, four pillars are usually described: autonomy—respect for a patient's right to self-determination; beneficence—the obligation to do good; nonmaleficence—the duty to not do bad; and justice—the obligation to treat all peoples equally. The beauty here is in the simplicity of these statements, but the challenges arrive in practice. Looking back to Dr. Niselle's statement, there are common intersection points between the law and medical ethics. For example, the ethical concept of autonomy is often associated in practice with the concepts of informed consent, privacy, and rights of access to one's own data. Beneficence is considered a key element of medical negligence law. Nonmaleficence is associated with criminal and negligence law, and justice is associated with legal aspects of nondiscrimination.

With respect to biomedical product development, the obligations and interplay of proper medical ethics varies slightly from the common scenarios of medical practice. First, the proper testing of medical products is subject to the concepts of ethical human subjects research, concepts that are built into the regulatory regime of the U.S. FDA and other federal regulators. In particular, ethics in research utilizes the same four pillars of medical ethics but also accounts for the many possible forms of conflict of interest that uniquely come into play in medical research.[6] For example, companies developing products obviously have significant financial interests in the success of the products, and bias must be managed appropriately. The same is potentially true for the clinicians who are leading the studies of these products and on down the line. Interestingly, the management of these potential conflicts can actually work against the patients within clinical studies.

The amorality of underregulated health technology

I have heard founders of startups and leadership with Silicon Valley refer to many technology-based business models as amoral, and I have found this to be true. The word usage here is important because the speakers in this case were using the word "amoral" to express moral neutrality, neither right nor wrong. But my take was more literal, that is, amoral means "lacking a sense of morality," which is not the same as being neutral. It is more reflective of a lack of education. This has been my experience, but I am not casting blame. It is more an observation of culture. Those of us who "grew up" in medicine and biomedical research are deeply steeped in the concepts of biomedical ethics early on and continuously via academic study, during the preparation and conduct of research, via repeated annual trainings, via direct experience, and via study and observation of the often-publicized mistakes of others. All of this is not true for many in Silicon Valley. Most of these folks grew up in traditional engineering, finance, and business school training that did not include anything about medical ethics. For example, the mission of the Massachusetts Institute of Technology (MIT) is to advance knowledge and educate students in science, technology, and other areas of scholarship that will best serve the nation and the world in the 21st century, as well as to generate, disseminate, and preserve knowledge, and to work with others to bring this knowledge to bear on the world's great challenges.[7] Noble to be sure, but nowhere in that mission does it mention "doing no harm," nor do engineers take anything similar to the Hippocratic oath, although the equivalent of the Hippocratic Oath has now been proposed for connected medical devices.[8] In practice, what I mostly have seen are ethical mistakes that are inevitable when the Silicon Valley approach of "move fast and break things" intersects with human subjects research.

Role of ethics in product regulation

Most of the ethics policies at the U.S. FDA deal with personal behavior, not with the rights or wrongs of medical products themselves. These policies exist to protect the agency, its employees, and consumers of the products regulated. The nature of these policies ranges from preventing criminal activity, such as bribery, to ensuring no inappropriate conflicts of interest, such as an FDA employee having decision influence over products from a sponsor in which they have a financial interest. Specifically, United States Code Title 18 contains the criminal conflict of interest statutes applicable to employees in the executive branch of the government. Included in Title 18 is a prohibition against solicitation or receipt of bribes; a prohibition against acting as an agent or attorney before the government; postemployment restrictions; a prohibition against participating in matters affecting personal financial interest; and a prohibition against receiving supplementation of salary as compensation for government service.[10] Although these elements of ethics are important, they are not our main focus. With respect to conflicts of interest, the relationships between medical product sponsors and the medical professionals involved in testing, evaluation, and prescribing of these products is also tightly regulated. In this specific case, by the Sunshine Act.[11] Unfortunately, the ethics of medical product regulation and the determination and evaluation of benefit risk are far less straightforward than the Sunshine Act. As will be discussed throughout the book, there can be a great tension or even dichotomy between medical innovation and the individual benefit-risk calculation for any given patient.

Patient rights and enablement

Listed within the four pillars is the concept of patient autonomy. The concept that patients have the right to make choices and to live by those choices is both simple and complex. Factors that influence and complicate are cultural, educational, situational, and individual. Starting with cultural, patient autonomy is primarily a principle of Western culture and can be quite different in the East or in communist or more autocratic nations. Education comes into play in many ways. First, clinicians are tasked with trying to ensure that medical conversations, especially those leading to decision-making, are adequately understood. Similarly, educational level must be considered by the consenting process for research procedures. Specifically, best practices for informed consent forms is that they be written at the sixth to eighth grade level to ensure understanding. Among the more common situational examples are instances when a patient may be unconscious or otherwise impaired and unable to agree to a diagnostic procedure, or cases in which the patient is an unattended minor or a psychologically impaired adult. Elements of individuality may include religion, sexual orientation, and other highly personal factors that could lead to less common personal preferences and boundaries that must be respected. So, in effect, every person is unique and likely has at least one personal situation or attribute that may not be obvious in a clinical or research situation but that must be respected.

One institutional approach to patient autonomy that is embedded within the healthcare lexicon in the United States is the Patient Bill of Rights. First adopted by the American Hospital Association (AHA) in 1973, the Patient Bill of Rights was developed with the expectation that hospitals and healthcare institutions would support these rights in the interest of delivering effective patient care.[12] The authors strongly suggest that medical technology innovators educate themselves on the Patient Bill of Rights. Indeed, mandatory training for key personnel would be even better.

Although all four pillars of medical ethics are relevant to digital health tools and transformation, patients' rights to privacy and to consent, to access and control over their own information, and to understanding partnerships of their healthcare institutions are especially important.

Medical privacy

As is explicitly stated multiple times within the Patient Bill of Rights, medical privacy is considered a basic and essential right in health care. Privacy is considered essential in health care for many reasons, chief among them the necessity to collect and utilize large amounts of personal data that uniquely identify the individual and, if exposed within the wrong contexts, could cause a spectrum of harms from embarrassment to financial and physical harm.

For example, many diseases, such as HIV, carry the risk of stigma. In the early days of HIV, tremendous stigma and fear were associated with the disease and still persist today. According to a United Nations AIDs report released in 2017, "When people living with, or at risk of, HIV are discriminated against in health-care settings, they go underground. This seriously undermines our ability to reach people with HIV testing, treatment and pre-vention services . . . Stigma and discrimination is an affront to human rights and puts the lives of people living with HIV and key populations in danger."[13] Worse, stigma can be a self-fulfilling prophecy, and it is not limited to life-threatening infectious diseases. The field of mental health offers another set of illnesses prone to stigmatization. According to the Mayo Clinic, the stigma of mental illness can lead to reluctance to seek help or treatment; lack of un-derstanding from family, friends, coworkers or others; fewer opportunities for work, school, or social activities; trouble finding housing; bullying, phys-ical violence, or harassment; health insurance that doesn't adequately cover mental illness treatment; and the belief that as an individual with mental ill-ness you will never succeed at certain challenges or be able to improve your situation.[14]

Beyond the risk of stigma, medical privacy is essential to prevent var-ious forms of discrimination. One important incarnation is the Genetic Information Nondiscrimination Act (GINA). According to the U.S. Department of Health and Human Services (HHS), GINA exists to protect individuals against health coverage and employment discrimination based on their genetic information. GINA is divided into two sections, or Titles. Title I of GINA prohibits discrimination based on genetic information in health coverage. Title II of GINA prohibits discrimination based on genetic infor-mation in employment.[15] There are several important things to note about GINA. First, it is an antidiscrimination law not a privacy law. The law does not prevent the sharing or exposure of sensitive genetic data. The law prevents specific uses of that data. According to the Electronic Frontier Foundation (EFF), a nongovernmental organization (NGO) dedicated to protecting civil liberties in the digital world, "GINA is essentially an anti-discrimination law that has nothing to do with privacy. It prevents group health and Medicare supplemental plans—but not life, disability, or long-term care plans—from using genetic information to discriminate against you when it comes to insur-ance."[16] Understanding distinctions such as this is critical to understanding privacy in the growing world of digital health. In short, not only are there myriad loopholes, new types of products that defy traditional regulatory regimens are being produced rapidly and regulators simply cannot keep up.

In the United States, the HIPAA privacy rule establishes national standards to protect individuals' protected health information (PHI), which includes medical records and other personal health information. The privacy rule applies to health plans, healthcare clearinghouses, and those healthcare providers who conduct certain healthcare transactions electronically.[17] However, at more than twenty years old, and conceived and implemented before the digital age, HIPAA is clearly underpowered to disincentivize many wrongdoers. The first of many structural gaps is the limitation in the applicability of HIPAA. According to the HIPAA journal, "HIPAA covers traditional healthcare organizations that perform electronic transactions—healthcare providers, health plans, and healthcare clearinghouses—as well as business associates of those organizations. The ONC points out that HIPAA Rules serve the healthcare industry well and ensure that appropriate controls are put in place to protect ePHI, but the scope of the legislation is limited. Many organizations that collect personal health information fall outside the scope of the HIPAA."[18] A large loophole exists where the same data elements that are explicitly protected when used by HIPAA covered entities are not protected from use by noncovered entities such as smart phone manufacturers, fitness devices, and the like. Practically, this means that supermarket loyalty card companies can trade and exchange personal health information, but two doctor's offices cannot do the same without legal risk. This is where the HIPAA Security Rule comes into play. According to the American Medical Association, "The HIPAA Security Rule requires physicians to protect patients' electronically stored, protected health information (known as "ePHI") by using appropriate administrative, physical and technical safeguards to ensure the confidentiality, integrity and security of this information."[19] These are exactly the reasons why a supermarket loyalty card can exchange or trade in information that doctors' offices and medical facilities cannot.

Privacy: Is health data the new blood?

In early 2019, Andrea Coravos and I published an open access article in the inaugural edition of *Lancet Digital Health* to probe issues surrounding data privacy, patient autonomy, data profiteering, and the attention economy. The piece riffs off an article published in *The Economist* in late 2018 declaring the world's most valuable resource was no longer oil but data.[20] The piece described the emergence of a highly lucrative data economy and warned that new antitrust legislation might be needed for greater governance of data. Comparing data to oil has been heavily criticized but that has not stopped use of the metaphor nor has it slowed the "gold rush"-like fervor with which many are trying to monetize personal health data (PHI) and/or personally identifiable information (PII).

The healthcare data economy is booming with hundreds of start-up companies looking to supposedly fix health care through innovative data, data tools, and technology products. In addition to these legitimate businesses, an equally booming shadow economy is driven by conventional wisdom that estimates the value of a medical record to be ten times the value of credit card data.

We are clearly seeing genuinely negative consequences to patients from the utilization of such data. The *Lancet* piece used the example of a continuous positive airway pressure (CPAP) device manufacturer who was sharing patient compliance data from these machines with insurers, who were subsequently denying patient claims on the basis of supposed adherence gaps.[21] In this case, a patient was denied coverage for accessories to the medical device because the device was transmitting usage data to the manufacturer without patient knowledge or consent. This raises many essential questions. Was the patient informed about the data transfer/sharing? Was the patient aware that "compliance" was being measured? Could power outages or Internet connectivity gaps skew the data? What are/were the patient rights in this case? What consumer protections exist regarding the collection, transmission, and use of this data in order to protect patients in the event of potential discrimination or data misuse?

As a potential solution, we suggest a model wherein patient data is granted the same legal status as physical bio-samples such as blood, by treating data as digital specimens. We propose a three-pronged strategy for avoiding harm and protecting the privacy of digital specimens. First, to enable regulation and protection, digital specimens must be properly categorized by at least three attributes: by data type or format; by level of permission such as consented, unconsented, informed but not consented; and by level of risk to the data donor. Practically, this could be implemented in a similar fashion to the special categories of data within Global Data Protection Regulations (GDPR). Implementation could help ensure that data is validated for quality and accuracy to avoid irresponsible, negligent, or methodologically invalid applications. Second, enabled by this categorization, new and more practically usable methods of consumer notification must replace or enhance the currently failing End User License Agreement model (also known as the, "agree to all the terms listed or you can't use this product" model).[22] Third, consumer protections must be put in place to inform and protect the public but also to notify in the case of a data breach and enable adequate penalties for privacy violations. In truth, we believe that these steps are the bare minimum that must be accomplished to include, engage, and protect digital specimen donors. We propose that digital specimens can be anything from medical records and DNA sequences to Amazon purchasing histories, given that any of these can be used to intrude upon privacy in ways that would be detrimental to patients and consumers. Applying the principle of digital specimens would turn the tables and place the burden of transparency, permission, and clarity onto the company wishing to utilize the data. All of this is essential in a space that is continually evolving and where policy does not appear to be catching up. Lastly, these protections are necessary, because there is currently no antidiscrimination law governing patient or personal data in the United States. The Genetic Non-Discrimination Act (GINA) is not a privacy law, but it does impose restrictions on uses that would be discriminatory. The same restrictions are needed for health and personal data.

There is no perfect privacy in the digital age

As discussed earlier, data is the currency of the digital economy and, although this itself is not necessarily harmful, the many possible misuses of the data can be quite harmful. Despite all the ethical and legal rationale for privacy, the fact is that there is no such thing as perfect personal privacy today unless an individual takes on a "survivalist-get-off-the-grid-and-live-underground-in-a-bunker-in-an-undisclosed-location," lifestyle, and even that person would likely be quite findable. That said, this situation is a great use of the expression, "Don't let the perfect be the enemy of the good." Just because perfect privacy is unrealistic, does not mean that we should not aim for as close to perfect as is reasonable. In fact, most people know this already. According to Marissa Lang, writing for the *San Francisco Chronicle* in 2017, "Just 12% of Americans and 9% of social media users report a 'very high level of confidence' that the government and tech companies can keep their personal information safe and secure, according to a Pew study from 2016."[23] It is good that people realize this, but what they may not realize are the potential impacts or harms. One important element of privacy in the digital age is disclosure. Although people may be aware that their data is not secure, what they need to know and understand is where is it going, to whom and for what uses, so transparent disclosure will be an essential component in any society without perfect privacy.

Disclosure is an example of what some would call a basic human right in the digital age. Following the Cambridge Analytica Scandal, the United Nations (UN) Human Rights Council requested that the High Commissioner of the UN prepare a report on the right to privacy in the digital age.[24,25] Beginning in 2014, Cambridge Analytica obtained data on 50 million Facebook users via means that deceived both the users and Facebook and are accused of manipulating information to sway elections, particularly the 2016 U.S. presidential election.[26] We will cover misinformation in greater detail later, but the simple version is that human opinion and emotion are deeply tied to an individual's belief systems and all of this is actually quite easily manipulated if you present "fake" data that is well-aligned with personal beliefs.

Getting back to the previously referenced UN Human Rights Council request, the result was a report published in August of 2018 titled, "The Right to Privacy in the Digital Age." The report is quite comprehensive and addresses privacy as a basic human right, as well as the responsibilities of government entities to protect it. Of course, when it comes to assaults on privacy, governments are frequent offenders. Among the government activities called out in the report are increased collection of the digital footprints of consumers, data and intelligence sharing across government and commercial entities, collection of biometric data (especially important in digital health), mass surveillance, offensive (as opposed to defensive) government hacking, legislative attempts to weaken encryption and anonymity, and cross-border access to data held by international businesses. In response, the UN recommends that nation states: put in adequate safeguards and oversight, create a framework to protect against undue interference, put in procedural safeguards against the interception of communications, ensure independent authorization and oversight, and ensure adequate transparency. Although all well-intentioned and articulated, it is easy to see how this is a bit like ordering the fox to guard the henhouse, with the principles of autonomy and independent authority being absolutely essential if any real safeguards are to evolve.

Lastly, it is important to not give up on privacy. Desensitization is defined as a process that diminishes emotional responsiveness to a negative, aversive, or positive stimulus after repeated exposure to it. This appears to be happening to many consumers. The endless list of data breaches and cybercrimes makes privacy seem impossible and makes the benefits of trying to remain private seem not worth the effort. What must be understood is that, unfortunately, things can get worse. Having to cancel a hacked credit card account and request a replacement is a relatively minor inconvenience to most, but events having a highly negative impact on a consumer credit score can be major inconveniences with significant financial and personal impacts, such as higher mortgage interest rates that can add tens of thousands of dollars to the cost of financing a home. Possibly more important than financial impact is the personal impact of stigma and the many possible associated harms previously discussed. Privacy can feel like a losing game, but we must remember that at least some of this is intentional. The industries making billions of dollars off of personal data certainly are not supportive of comprehensive privacy regulation. It truly is analogous to expecting the tobacco industry to support antinicotine laws. They will fight against the basic human rights of digital privacy, and we must not give up and let them win.

Data ownership

An important aspect of privacy is data ownership. There are many definitions of it and each carries authority, along with limitations and responsibilities. Starting with the word "ownership," many feel that individuals are the owners of their data and, therefore, should have complete control and be the only ones who can permit access, sharing, or use. Although logical, these concepts start to break down almost immediately upon examination. Take home ownership or automobile ownership, as examples of other assets people own. Along with clear rights, authority, and privilege, there are obligations and liabilities that can be considered downsides. For example, if someone is injured on another's property, the owners may be liable. Well, what about a cancer patient in a Facebook group with poor password practices that is hacked and then serves as an attack vector for others on the social network? The World Wide Web is very much like a physical crowd, wherein the actions of one person, intentional or accidental, can put others at risk. Beyond attempting to understand the basic concepts of ownership, the next issue to address is the concept of stakeholders who believe they have an ownership stake. The list includes doctors, hospitals' electronic medical record (EMR) and technology vendors, payers, and even the state in which the records reside.

Any discussion of who technically owns electronic health record data can quickly become complex. According to *Medical Economics*, back in 2014, "Who owns patient data in an electronic health record (EHR)? It's a simple question with a complex answer. No longer confined to the shelves of a physician's office, patient data is now shared and used by a myriad of organizations across healthcare: Other physicians and health systems, the EHR vendor, payers, and researchers, not to mention patients themselves. While primary care physicians often originate the medical record, the resulting data are not theirs alone. The implication? The traditional concept of ownership is unraveling as patient data migrates away from paper charts and takes up residence in the cloud. Experts now counsel physicians against the concept of data ownership entirely. Instead, they encourage physicians to consider themselves "stewards" of the data within their possession and administrative control."[27] Interestingly, like many things in technology and medicine, ownership may have been determined more by precedent set by litigation than by legislation.

An excellent resource for determining legal data ownership is the "Health Information and the Law" project run by George Washington University and the Robert Wood Johnson Foundation, which has done a superb job compiling and presenting data ownership by state as well as details on underlying litigation and legislation. There is a wealth of interesting facts. First, the only state in which patients legally own their EMR data is New Hampshire.[28] Some 19 states have laws stating the electronic medical record is the property of the hospital and or physician; and it must be noted that if a hospital is publicly owned and operated by a state, then the data is likely considered owned by that state. In the remaining states, no laws identified confer specific ownership or property right to medical records. In Massachusetts, my home state, there are laws stating that physicians must keep and maintain medical records for at least seven years, hospitals must keep and maintain records for 20 years, physicians must provide patients the opportunity to inspect their records, and public health officials are permitted access to all these records in order to monitor and prevent the spread of disease. This last issue being especially important in infectious disease outbreaks such as COVID-19.

The next element of data "ownership" to consider is use. To many, this is really the crux of data ownership. In many ways and to many patients, who technically "owns" their medical data is less important than how that data is being used. According to the Office of the National Coordinator for Health Information Technology (ONC), as of 2017, some 94% of hospitals were using medical record data to support processes that inform clinical practices.[29] Specifically, EHR data is most commonly used by hospitals to support quality improvement (82%), monitor patient safety (81%), and measure organization performance (77%). These uses appear ethically, medically, and scientifically valid, and the fact that ONC is keeping track is also a bonus. Where things start to slide quickly off the rails is when the data start to be exploited for additional uses that do not align nearly as congruently with the data ownership and/or stewardship laws.

A booming data economy is built around secondary uses of health data, and privacy and ethics concerns abound. A great many private companies have popped up to trade in health and other personal information, such as consumer-spending data. Most claim benevolent intentions, but, as we have seen via high-profile scandals such as the previously discussed Cambridge Analytica mess, many of these companies are simply seeking profit. Add a business model of profiteering on data to the amorality of Silicon Valley culture and the result is a predictable mess. According to Craig Klugman, writing for Bioethics.net in late 2018,

> Using patients' medical data for anything other than their care or quality improvement is unethical as it violates trust. Patients share their private information (i.e. secrets) because their doctors have a duty to maintain confidentiality and to only use the data to treat, diagnose, and improve care. In other words, patients share

their secrets with the expectation that this knowledge will be used only to help them. They trust that their secrets will remain confidential because physicians and health care entities have a fiduciary responsibility to do so. However, these private companies and data brokers do not have fiduciary responsibilities toward patients, especially if there is some effort at anonymizing the records."[30]

It is also important to note that deidentification often can be foiled; studies have shown this time and time again by easily reidentifying records that were supposedly deidentified in a foolproof manner.

Having taken all of that into consideration, it must be noted that many of these companies believe they are doing a public good and that there should be an ethical obligation for patients to share data to help themselves and others get better care. On certain levels, these arguments do hold up. A Pew Research survey and study in 2016 found that just more than half, 52%, of Americans feel that health-data sharing was acceptable.[31] Interestingly, 62% of individuals over the age of 50 felt data sharing was OK, but only 45% of those aged 18–45 felt the same. It would be interesting to know why this is. Specifically, is there an element of cyber awareness for the younger generations that impacts this thinking? If so, they are probably right.

The fact is there have been more examples of scandals over secondary data use than public success stories. It is difficult to believe that organizations lacking deep expertise in data science, biostatistics, and bioethics are capable of producing high-quality research. Another case for caveat emptor for sure but more of a warning for institutions than individuals. Public trust is low and falling quickly due to high-profile and controversial deals such as the deal that Sloan Kettering made with an artificial intelligence company or the Ascension Health deal with Google.[32,33] Both of these deals sparked outrage and concern regarding privacy and patient rights, but neither, conceptually, is inherently bad for patients. The issues are of autonomy and the ethics of profiteering, and it can be impossible to say upfront which such deals are likely to produce value to patients in the long run. Hence, the benefit-risk calculus is hard to determine at the time the deals are announced or discovered.

Lastly, it is important to note that there are definitely two sides to this story. The fact that the Pew Study showed 52% approval of medical-data sharing shows a fairly even split in the populace, and we must remain vigilant that both sides and points of view are respected. It is feared that scandals such as the above will make healthcare institutions more concerned with liability and therefore conservative and hesitant to innovate. This is clearly not great for patients either. The devil is in the details and, in these cases, following traditional routes and practices, such as solid IRB oversight and comprehensive patient consent, can pave the way for innovation without as much liability. This is what can be so frustrating about this data market and the players. In many cases if not most, simply taking the appropriate and well-known steps in the conduct of ethical human subjects research would enable the study and protect against liability and reputational risk. Why not do it but do it right? Is it ignorance, arrogance, or malfeasance? We have seen all three. We can hope that clear best practices will be the path of the future, as well as make the most sense from a business perspective.

It is also important to understand that medical privacy is not really separate from consumer privacy. The 18 HIPAA-recognized identifiers of personal health information (PHI) are:

- Name
- Address (all geographic subdivisions smaller than state, including street address, city/county, and zip code)
- All elements (except years) of dates related to an individual (including birthdate, admission date, discharge date, date of death, and exact age if over 89)
- Telephone numbers
- Fax number
- E-mail address
- Social Security Number
- Medical record number
- Health plan beneficiary number
- Account number
- Certificate or license number
- Vehicle identifiers and serial numbers, including license plate numbers
- Device identifiers and serial numbers
- Web URL
- Internet Protocol (IP) Address
- Finger or voice print
- Photographic image—Photographic images are not limited to images of the face.
- Any other characteristic that could uniquely identify the individual.[34]

A quick look at this list confirms that only a few of these are unique to medical records, and most are just personal information that is typically referred to outside of medical contexts as personally identifiable information (PII). There are several important points to note. First, most of this data is available on individuals many times over outside of medical contexts, hence, there is barely a gray line between medical and nonmedical personal data. Second, per the discussion of the ease of reidentifying deidentified data, with modest effort this exogenous data can be linked with PHI to uniquely reidentify individuals. Third, the combination of PII and PHI, as well as the dozens of other data types each of us creates, is considered extremely high value in medicine and within the secondary data economy.

Can there be personalized medicine without surveillance?

Lastly, one of the promises of the genomic and digital age is personalized medicine. The National Cancer Institute defines personalized medicine as "A form of medicine that uses information about a person's genes, proteins, and environment to prevent, diagnose, and treat disease. In cancer, personalized medicine uses specific information about a person's tumor to help diagnose, plan treatment, find out how well treatment is working, or make a prognosis.[35] Considering this definition, the process described of "using specific information about a person's tumor" clearly defines data usage that uniquely identifies a person in a highly specific manner. As a patient of personalized cancer care myself, the periods between treatment and scanning for changes in my tumors is typically referred to as "watchful waiting" or surveillance. Put simply, the doctors are watching me over time. This is very close to the most common uses of the word "surveillance." Of course, I accept this decrease in personal privacy because the benefits of knowing my cancer is under control is an absolute necessity for my family and me, but it is a trade-off. Similarly, almost all of the promises of digital health will involve privacy trade-offs. As we will discuss later, real-time sensors, patient diaries, new diagnostics all will be tracked in a manner that can only be described as surveillance.

References

1. Wright VC. Laser Surgery: Using the Carbon Dioxide Laser. *Canadian Medical Association Journal* 1982. 126(9):1035–1039.
2. Akhtar N, F Ansar, MS Baig, and A Abbas. Airway Fires during Surgery: Management and Prevention. *Journal of Anaesthesiology, Clinical Pharmacology* 2016. 32(1):109–111.
3. Murray PM. The History of Informed Consent. *Iowa Orthopaedic Journal* 1990. 10:104–109.
4. U.S. FDA. FDA Warns Against Use of Energy-Based Devices to Perform Vaginal "Rejuvenation" or Vaginal Cosmetic Procedures: FDA Safety Communication. 2018, July. Accessed November 2019. https://www.fda.gov/medical-devices/safety-communications/ fda-warns-against-use-energy-based-devices-perform-vaginal-rejuvenation-or-vaginal-cosmetic

5. Niselle P. Essential Learning: Law and Ethics. Medicalprotection.org. 2019, January. Accessed November 2019. https://www.medicalprotection.org/uk/articles/essential-learning-law-and-ethics

6. Avasthi A, A Ghosh, S Sarkar, and S Grover. Ethics in Medical Research: General Principles with Special Reference to Psychiatry Research. *Indian Journal of Psychiatry* 2013. 55(1):86–91. doi:10.4103/0019-5545.105525

7. MIT. Mission. MIT Facts. Accessed November 2019. https://web.mit.edu/facts/mission.html

8. Woods B, A Coravos, and JD Corman. The Case for a Hippocratic Oath for Connected Medical Devices: Viewpoint. *Journal Medical Internet Research* 2019. 21(3):e12568. doi:10.2196/12568

9. U.S. FDA. Ethics Laws and Regulations. 2019, May. Accessed August 2019. https://www.fda.gov/about-fda/ethics/ethics-laws-and-regulations

10. Hwong A, and L Lehmann. Putting the Patient at the Center of the Physician Payment Sunshine Act. *Health Affairs Blog.* 2012, June 13.

11. American Hospital Association. Patient Bill of Rights. 1992. Accessed October 2019. http://www.qcc.cuny.edu/SocialSciences/ppecorino/MEDICAL_ETHICS_TEXT/Chapter_6_Patient_Rights/Readings_The%20Patient_Bill_of_Rights.htm

12. UNAIDS. Press Release. UNAIDS Warns that HIV-related Stigma and Discrimination Is Preventing People from Accessing HIV Services. 2017, October 3. Accessed December 2019. https://www.unaids.org/en/resources/presscentre/pressreleaseandstatementarchive/2017/october/20171002_confronting-discrimination

13. Mayo Clinic Staff. Mental Health: Overcoming the Stigma of Illness. 2017, May 24. Accessed December 2019. https://www.mayoclinic.org/diseases-conditions/mental-illness/in-depth/mental-health/art-20046477

14. U.S. HHS. Health Information Privacy: Genetic Information. 2017, June 16. Accessed November 2019. https://www.hhs.gov/hipaa/for-professionals/special-topics/genetic-information/index.html

15. Electronic Frontier Foundation. Genetic Information Privacy. Accessed November 2019. https://www.eff.org/issues/genetic-information-privacy

16. U.S. HHS. The HIPAA Privacy Rule. 2015 April 16. Accessed December 2019. https://www.hhs.gov/hipaa/for-professionals/privacy/index.html

17. HIPAA Journal Staff. Large Privacy and Security Gaps at Non-HIPAA Covered Entities Highlighted by ONC Report. 2016, July 20. Accessed September 2019. https://www.hipaajournal.com/large-privacy-security-gaps-non-hipaa-covered-entities-onc-report-3512/

18. AMA. HIPAA Security Rule and Risk Analysis. Accessed December 2019. https://www.ama-assn.org/practice-management/hipaa/hipaa-security-rule-risk-analysis

19. Regulating the Internet Giants: The World's Most Valuable Resource Is No Longer Oil, But Data. *The Economist.* 2017, May 6. https://www.economist.com/leaders/2017/05/06/the-worlds-most-valuable-resource-is-no-longer-oil-but-data

20. Perakslis E, and A Coravos. Is Health-Care Data the New Blood? *Lancet Digital Health* 2019. 1(1):PE8–E9.

21. Allen M. You Snooze, You Lose: How Insurers Dodge the Cost of Popular Sleep Apnea Devices. National Public Radio, Washington, DC. 2018, November 21. Accessed December 2019. https://www.npr.org/sections/healthshots/2018/11/21/669751038/you-snoozeyou-lose-how-insurers-dodge-the-costs-of-popularsleep-apnea-devices

22. Obar JA, and A Oeldorf-Hirsch. The Biggest Lie on the Internet: Ignoring the Privacy Policies and Terms of Service Policies of Social Networking Services. *Information Communication and Society* 2016. 2016:1–20.

23. Lang M. There Is No Such Thing as True Privacy in the Digital Age. *Government Technology* 2017, March 10. Accessed November 2019. https://www.govtech.com/security/There-is-No-Such-Thing-as-True-Privacy-in-the-Digital-Age.html

24. United Nations General Assembly. The Right to Privacy in the Digital Age. 2014, June 30. Downloaded July 2019. https://www.ohchr.org/en/issues/digitalage/pages/digitalageindex.aspx

25. Privacy International. The Next Frontier of the Right to Privacy in the Digital Age. 2018, October 2. Accessed November 2019. https://privacyinternational.org/blog/2317/next-frontier-right-privacy-digital-age

26. Ingram D. Factbox: Who is Cambridge Analytica and What Did It Do? *Reuters Technology News*. 2018, March 19. Accessed September 2019. https://www.reuters.com/article/us-facebook-cambridge-analytica-factbox/factbox-who-is-cambridge-analytica-and-what-did-it-do-idUSKBN1GW07F

27. Medical Economics. The Battle Over EHR Patient Data. 2014, October 21. Accessed May 2019. https://www.medicaleconomics.com/editors-choice-me/battle-over-ehr-patient-data

28. HealthInfoLaw. Who Owns Medical Records: 50 State Comparison. 2012. Accessed October 2019. http://www.healthinfolaw.org/comparative-analysis/who-owns-medical-records-50-state-comparison

29. Parasrampuria S, and J Henery. Health IT Data Brief. Hospital's Use of Electronic Health Records Data: 2015–2017. Office of the National Coordinator for Health IT. 2019 April. No. 46.

30. Klugman C. Hospitals Selling Patient Records To Data Brokers: A Violation of Patient Trust and Autonomy. Bioethics.net. 2018, December 12. Accessed October 2019. http://www.bioethics.net/2018/12/hospitals-selling-patient-records-to-data-brokers-a-violation-of-patient-trust-and-autonomy/

31. Snell E. Majority of Americans Say Health Data Sharing Acceptable. *Patient Privacy News* 2016, January 20. Accessed October 2019. https://healthitsecurity.com/news/majority-of-americans-say-health-data-sharing-acceptable

32. Ornstein C, and K Thomas. Sloan Kettering's Cozy Deal with Start-Up Ignites a New Uproar. *New York Times*. 2018, September 20. Accessed October 2019. https://www.nytimes.com/2018/09/20/health/memorial-sloan-kettering-cancer-paige-ai.html

33. Davis J. Google Ascension Partnership Fuels Overdue HIPAA Privacy Debate. *HealthITSecurity*. 2019, December 20. Accessed December 2019. https://healthitsecurity.com/news/google-ascension-partnership-fuels-overdue-hipaa-privacy-debate

34. Gellman R. The Deidentification Dilemma: A Legislative and Contractual Proposal. Fpf.org. 2010, July 12. Accessed July 2019. https://fpf.org/wp-content/uploads/2010/07/The_Deidentification_Dilemma.pdf

35. National Cancer Institute. NCI Dictionary of Cancer Terms. Accessed December 2019. https://www.cancer.gov/publications/dictionaries/cancer-terms/def/personalized-medicine

4

The Evolution of Digital Technologies in Health Care

During the summer of 1985, I worked as a biomedical engineering technology (BMET) intern at a small but well-to-do suburban hospital just west of Boston, Massachusetts. I was excited, honored, and appreciative to have been selected out of my class in engineering school given that most of my friends also had applied for this one spot.

A brief overview of clinical technology in the mid-1980s

The hospital was a fascinating maze of technology in multiple dimensions. The physical layout was sprawling, because the hospital was founded as a cottage hospital in 1881 and had grown room by room at first but eventually floor by floor and wing by wing. The biomedical engineering shop (BMET) was located in a maintenance wing that was central from the standpoint of the physical campus but well away from patient areas. We were co-located with all of the trade and maintenance areas. Outside our door were the electrical and mechanical workshops, as well as the plumbing, carpentry, general maintenance, and machine areas. Our BMET shop was small but fully modern for the day. There was a desk for the lead technician, Jim, a workbench for the other full-time technician, Victor, and a worktable in the middle where I was seated. Unlike the rest of the maintenance wing, our shop had a door and the ability to insulate ourselves and the equipment we were servicing from noise, dust, or "borrowing." The only area of the hospital for which we were not responsible was radiology and nuclear medicine, because those highly specialized areas had dedicated expert support.

Outside of our immediate area was a fascinating and foreign land to me. Each area was physically structured for highly specific technological functioning. The patient floors were open and bright with private and double rooms equipped with basic equipment for patient care. This included electric

Digital Health. Eric D. Perakslis and Martin Stanley, Oxford University Press (2021). © Oxford University Press.
DOI: 10.1093/oso/9780197503133.003.0004

adjustable beds, medical gas ports and fixtures, wall-mounted mercury-column blood pressure manometers and cuffs, nurse call buttons, and televisions. I list all this equipment because this is where I started, that first summer: going room to room inspecting, cleaning, and servicing every piece of equipment in each of the 200-plus med-surg beds.

The primary electronic medical equipment annual safety testing requirement of the Joint Commission on Accreditation of Hospitals (JCAH) at that time was electrical safety testing. In short, this testing seeks to minimize the risk of electric shock to patients or healthcare workers. The main variables were ground resistance and current leakage, and these were measured by a simple lunch-box-sized tester. You plugged the piece of equipment in, pressed a few buttons, and if the numbers were within specifications, the device passed. There was also a visual inspection for frayed wires, damaged power cord caps, loose cord cap tongs, and a host of other similar elements. If the instrument passed, an inspection sticker was applied and the details logged in logbooks, which were organized by unit/floor/ward/room and equipment type. If the instrument did not pass, most repairs could be made onsite, but if the room being inspected was occupied, the equipment needed to be swapped out. We could not do bed safety checks on beds containing patients, so it was an iterative process working with the nursing and housekeeping staff to eventually inspect all beds on each floor.

It should be said that a hospital environment is not kind to simple or complex electrical equipment. Beds are moved around frequently, and power chords are dropped, crushed, and torn. Fluids are everywhere and not highly compatible with electronics. Equipment gets dropped, smashed, moved, lost, and buried under all manner of things mundane and messy. The most common repairs were to replace power cord caps, often the site of ground resistance, and frayed cords. Nurse-call cords and wired TV remote controls were constantly in need of cleaning and rewiring, and the older hospital beds could occasionally have stray current leakage that had to be chased down.

The other most common task was the cleaning and inspection of the wall-mounted, mercury-filled sphygmomanometers, which is the technical term for blood pressure gauges. These simple devices remain the gold standard in blood pressure measurement but are being phased out due to environmental concerns around the use of mercury. These concerns did not exist in 1985. Indeed, we essentially played in the stuff all day long. The most common issue with these devices was oxidation of the mercury that would collect at the top of the mercury column and interfere with the accuracy of the blood pressure reading. The calibration procedure was to swap each device, one-by-one, with a newly calibrated unit, bring the unit to the shop, drain the mercury into a bowl, clean the graduated glass tube, filter the mercury through a conical filter, not unlike a paper coffee filter, return the cleaned mercury to the device, and perform a quick operational verification procedure (OVP), typically by comparing the pressure on the device with a single pressurized standard. All of the above was accomplished using a minimum of safety gear, gloves and a mask on an open table in a cramped shop, and I did this hundreds of times over that summer. Who knew you shouldn't play with that much mercury . . . ?

Beyond the medical-surgical patient floors, was the really cool stuff, and I couldn't wait to learn about all of it. The specialization and intricate integration of physical rooms, medical equipment, and specialized diagnostics and care appeared infinite, but I wanted to understand it all. From the clicks and beeps of all the highly specialized vital signs monitoring and life support equipment in the intensive care unit (ICU), cardiac care unit (CCU), anesthesia, surgical recovery ward, and labor and delivery (L&D) to the horribly scary and painful looking equipment of the cystoscopy (urinary tract visualization) and colonoscopy areas to the specialized surgery suites, emergency ward, and birthing rooms, I took it all in hungrily over that first summer. Beyond the luck of landing the position, my exposure opportunity was significant given that there were only three of us in the department, including the director who was able to do technical work only about half the time. His expertise was digital and analogue electronics while Victor's was pulmonary and other pneumatic equipment. I got to be the grunt for both of them, charged with all things mundane, and I could not have been more fortunate.

The technology of the day differed less from that of today than might be expected. The basics of hospital rooms and the purpose and specialization of the diagnostic and treatment areas remain quite similar. There was "Wi-Fi," in the form of basic telemetry, wherever useful, such as in the cardiac care stepdown unit where recovering patients were encouraged to be up and walking. The critical care areas such as the ICU and CCU had an array of bedside vital-signs monitoring equipment that was repeated, via hardwire, at the nursing stations. Anesthesia stations were already self-contained life support units with significant electronic and medical gas functionality. Surgical suites varied greatly from very basic more or less "no-tech," general purpose rooms to highly specialized laser surgery and cystoscopy suites. The labor and delivery area was, probably, the most modern for the day. This hospital was renowned for prenatal and postnatal care and had invested accordingly. There were "natural" birthing rooms that resembled a well-furnished home bedroom or hotel room with the exception of the significant and powerful medical machinery that was hidden from sight within the cabinetry to be ready at a moment's notice if needed. Down the hall were two fully equipped operating suites for planned or unplanned cesarean section procedures.

With the exception of the specific telemetry-enabled areas previously described, for the most part, the electronic equipment was stand-alone and not networked. This required the constant and contiguous presence of clinicians and technicians during the course of diagnostic and interventional procedures. Indeed, most of the equipment was also single function. Most electrocardiography (ECG) monitors were 3-lead, stand-alone lunchbox-sized units with separate and isolated AC power and proprietary leads and sensors. Some of the more advanced units were modular in that one large cathode-ray screen could display data from multiple data collection modules such as ECG, blood pressure, cardiac output, and others. From the standpoint of operational verification, service, and repair, these were our favorites, because we could swap out modules quickly in case of problems without having to remove the entire unit off the wall or station. The other prevalent element was that much of the equipment was analog or utilized analog components. For example, most pressure gauges were physical devices and still are today. Beyond this though, just like the automobiles of the time, many parts were mechanical (think carburetor vs. electronic fuel-injection). Mechanical machines generate heat and often contain parts that wear over time due to friction; this process often results in dust and dirt accumulation, which requires cleaning and exacting physical calibration.

Although the purpose, equipment, and function of most areas would be recognizable and familiar today, the operating models were indeed quite different. Most strikingly, at that time, universal blood and body precautions were just being introduced and were far from fully understood or utilized.[1] It was not uncommon at all to see technicians remove their gloves for better feel when dealing with a difficult venipuncture. In general, however, practices were good. People used common sense and changed gloves when going from room-to-room, etc., but all this would change, as, in January of 1985, the Centers for Disease Control and Prevention (CDC) updated the case definition of acquired immunodeficiency syndrome (AIDS) to note that the disease was caused by a single virus and to introduce the first provisional guidelines for blood screening.[2] This time period also saw the earliest peaks of AIDS hysteria and panic, which was my earliest exposure to the complex interdependencies of social issues and medicine. In September of 1985, my summer internship at the hospital was ending, but my performance had yielded a part-time job offer that would lead, several years later, to my first full-time job. Also, that September, *Time* magazine published a piece on AIDS hysteria. Titled "The New Untouchables," it detailed the growing anxiety, panic, and discrimination that was to come.[3] All of this piqued my curiosity and started my ongoing interest in infection prevention and control. Solid information was sparse, however, and the hospital library, a favorite place of mine, only contained one book on AIDS. I recall that the title was something like, "AIDS and Other Diseases of Homosexual Men," although despite my best efforts, I have been unable to find references to this book anywhere on the Internet. As you can guess, this book presented a very specific point of view that was also an important education for me on the stigma of disease.

Ensuring medical safety

As stated earlier, my very first set of tasks was to learn and execute procedures intended to ensure the safety of the equipment for patients and staff. This not only taught me the importance of safety in medical care environments, it also revealed how many things could go wrong and how quickly, or how slowly and silently things could go wrong. Let us start with devices as simple as hospital beds. Between January 1, 1985 and January 1, 2013, the U.S. Food and Drug Administration (FDA) received reports of 901 incidents of patients caught, trapped, entangled, or strangled in hospital beds. The reports included 531 deaths, 151 nonfatal injuries, and 220 cases where staff intervened to prevent an injury. Most of the affected patients were frail, elderly, or confused.[4] Guard rails were meant to prevent patients from falling out of bed and to assist patients. Getting in and out of bed often can be the cause of entrapment. Walking from room to room day after day doing electrical safety checks on beds never felt mundane, because it was too easy to picture a hospital bed, containing one of the many patients I met that summer, going up in flames due to an electrical issue that I should have detected and a fire I should have prevented.

Medical safety was a constant theme and ensuring medical safety entailed a unique set of requirements for each equipment type in each setting, although infection prevention and control, as well as electrical safety were universal. It is truly impressive how frequently expensive and complex medical equipment can be hit by all manner of splats and splatters from all manner of fluids. Fortunately, we seldom found such equipment in active use, rather, we most frequently would find unexpected gifts outside our door, on our workbenches, or in equipment storage rooms that were adjacent to or within each ward. We seldom knew what the fluid was or exactly what had happened. We were careful and thorough, but, as stated earlier, this was before universal body fluid precautions. By comparison to today, therefore, we were probably not careful enough with respect to protecting ourselves. The equipment got the full treatment though and was cleaned thoroughly inside and out. Any damaged parts or parts that could not be completely cleaned were swapped out and replaced prior to OVP and return to service. I had no understanding of the actual quantitative risks of high-touch hospital equipment. Since then studies have shown that surface disinfection, which is essentially what we always did, is helpful in decreasing the presence of infectious agents on equipment, but the specific types of disinfection still require further study, especially with respect to the efficacy of disinfection methods on specific pathogens such as MRSA, *c-dif*, and VRE, and the fact that not all equipment types carry equal risk of exposure.[5,6] Indeed, every piece of equipment we touched, inspected, or serviced received a thorough wipe down and cleaning, including the Q-tip treatment in every crevice or groove, which was often quite entertaining to the nurses observing us.

Electrical safety was similarly uniform across all wards and equipment types. If there was an AC power chord on the device, electrical safety was performed. The operational verification, along with additional, more-specialized safety checks were unique to each type of equipment, and this required and involved many new and exotic types of tools. Need to know if a cardiac defibrillator is delivering the correct amount of charge? There is a specific tested that measures the electrical current output. Need to know the electrical conductivity of the floor in each operating room? You attach metal cups to the soles of your properly covered shoes and walk around the room generating current between your own two feet by spinning a hand-cranked generator and measuring the resulting conductivity. Proper functioning of ECG machines can be determined via a dedicated simulator or by personally wearing ECG leads and testing the unit on yourself—in a pinch. The exact flow rates and composition of anesthetic gasses on each anesthesia station must be frequently measured and calibrated. On those days, it was best to avoid driving and have a ride home . . . .

As I learned and practiced, I was slowly given increasingly more complex equipment to study, along with more rope to hang myself, and I was soon put to trial by fire. Toward the end of that first summer, unexpected events found me alone, holding down the entire shop without technical supervision or support. This was never supposed to happen, but it did. I was wearing my boss' pager and on call 24 hours a day for about a week. I stayed late and came in early, and I tried to handle everything I could. I survived and learned a great deal from the experience.

Shortly after both my supervisors and mentors had returned, my director asked me to go for a walk with him. We strolled to the equipment room that was adjacent to the ICU. When he opened the door and turned on the lights, the room was quite full of equipment and much of it looked familiar. Most of the equipment had notes on it and many were not kind. Phrases such as "STILL BROKEN!" written in bright red marker were most common, although there were also some artful and poetic curses included on many. The equipment was also familiar, given that I was looking at much of my work from the week I was home alone. Expecting I was about to be fired, I was completely unprepared for the conversation that followed. Instead, Jim congratulated me for a great summer and asked if I would like a part-time job during the school year. I was very confused as I stared around at a room full of embarrassment. He then went on to explain that I never should have been put in that position in the first place, and that he had received only glowing feedback on my efforts during that time. Yes, certainly I had made mistakes, but they were not mine, they were the collective responsibility of the team, and we would fix them all together. This remains one of the most profound leadership lessons of my career, and I will always be deeply thankful to Jim for the gift he gave me that day.

In most ways, the clinical environment of today is quite similar to that of the mid-1980s. When it comes to typical hospital rooms, there are far fewer cords, because many devices now use wireless connections. Vital-signs monitoring hasn't changed much, but the way that vital signs and all other parts of patient care are documented, directly into an electronic medical record system, has been a massive change. In addition, many devices have been miniaturized and are wireless but now share networks with many other devices.

Electronic health records and the wired clinic

Probably the greatest single technology change in the clinics since the 1980s has been the wholesale adoption of electronic medical records (EMRs). The significance and complexity of this topic warrants its own chapter and is covered in detail later. For now, it is important to understand that the transformation from paper to electronic records in the clinic was driven by massive federal investment via the American Recovery and Reinvestment Act (ARRA) and that, despite great progress, significant challenges remain. The primary controversy and criticism being the immense amount of data entry, which some claim has turned clinicians into data-entry clerks. Further, many feel that it is even more difficult to get data out of these systems. Beyond the usability challenges, the ongoing costs, data processing and management burdens, and the disruption to patient-clinician interaction are all fundamental elements of

EHRs that must be optimized before there will be wide-scale recognition of the benefits of this particular clinical technology transformation.

The other significant change in the technical environment of hospitals is the pervasive use of data networking. Back in the day, patient networks were used in a limited matter in specialty settings, such as the ICU and cardiac care stepdown units, but there was no Internet to which to connect these isolated networks. They were physically isolated and, therefore, secure by air gap, which was not all that secure, but the level of threat was far less back then. This is not the case today, a fact that should be of great concern. In the first *Jurassic Park* movie, Jeff Goldblum's character made this profound (for Hollywood) statement about humans manufacturing dinosaurs: "You were so busy proving you could do something that you never stopped to consider if you should." There's a lesson here for today's technology innovators, and it is time for us all to seriously consider which patient care and monitoring devices are worth the risk of connecting to the Internet.

Cyber security in health care will always be difficult, given that medical care and practice require instant access to data and enabling diagnostic and treatment technologies. Healthcare workers require high availability systems and don't have the luxury of time to manage multifactor authentication and complex encryption solutions as they move from room to room, and patient to patient. Yet one important and overlooked strategy in this is for medical device and technology vendors to apply solid benefit-risk frameworks when deciding whether a medical device needs to be directly connected to the Internet or a local data network.

For example, connecting an implantable pacemaker to the Internet allows for software updates to be automated, the device's performance to be monitored, and even the patient's physiology to be tracked. This functionality confers clear benefits to the device manufacturer from the standpoint of quality control and risk management. It also offers potential benefits for patients, but what are the corresponding risks? Could hackers disrupt the device? Could loss of signal lead to a perception of device malfunction, possibly leading to unnecessary procedures? What about patient privacy? Technologically, these types of attacks are clearly possible, but how do we calculate the medical risk-benefit ratio? Unlike hospital-acquired infections, adverse drug reactions, and other well-quantified models of medical risk-benefit, we have no clear or common frameworks for cyber threats in health care. Yet with U.S. hospitals currently having on average 10–15 connected devices per bed, we desperately need them.[7]

Interestingly, while calculating the risk-benefit ratio of implantable pacemakers and other medical devices is complex, we are increasingly encountering another kind of situation where the tradeoffs are clear. More and more, we are bombarded with marketing and pop-science content promoting gadgets, appliances, and devices with Internet connectivity. Even if they are not medical devices and serve no purpose in the care of patients, in the Internet of things (IoT) all these appliances and gadgets have the potential to compromise healthcare systems.

In 2017, the IoT brought us IoT coffee machines that took down factory networks; IoT fish tanks that were used to hack a casino; hackers seizing control of everything from automobiles to Hover scooters; and the list goes on and on.[8,9,10] While an Internet-connected toaster appears convenient and harmless, the real danger is not the device itself, but—as in most of the cases above—the potential for that device to be exploited to gain entry to and attack or exploit a connected network.

Using the infection control metaphor I used in a *BMJ* Opinion piece, connected devices are infection vectors, and their chains of transmission can be complex.[11] For example, consider a grade-school child who connects their laptop or phone to the wireless network at their school and at home. Now assume that the child has a parent who connects their phone to that same home network, as well as to the hospital network where they are employed. You now have a viable chain of transmission from a public elementary school to a hospital network. Not only is this chain of access viable, it is actually attractive, because the hackers can target any institution indirectly, which provides a layer of misdirection that can shield their actions from investigation. This happens every day.

Where are the essential benefits to offset the cyber risks of IoT devices and appliances? How "wired" should even the most modern hospitals be? Healthcare workers, administrators, and engineers have the opportunity to exert control over cyber threats within their environments by simply keeping these things in mind when managing the physical clinical environment.

Yet the connected world we live in means that these questions aren't just confined to medical technology or devices used in a healthcare setting. The simple truth is that cyber risk decreases as the number of connected devices (endpoints) is decreased.[12] Perhaps we should be thinking of assessing the medical risk-benefit ratio of any device that is part of a chain of access to a healthcare system.

There is no doubt that technological advances are improving health care, but they bring with them complex and unexpected new risks as well as significant cost implications. The difference between great success and spectacular failure may simply lie in careful execution and proactive thought. It is clear that new models and frameworks of benefit risk are needed to incorporate these highly complex new modalities of risk.

References

1. CDC. Perspectives in Disease Prevention and Health Promotion Update: Universal Precautions for Prevention of Transmission of Human Immunodeficiency Virus, Hepatitis B Virus, and Other Bloodborne Pathogens in Health-Care Settings. 1988. 37(24):377–388.
2. HIV.gov. A Timeline of HIV and AIDS. Accessed May 2019. https://www.hiv.gov/hiv-basics/overview/history/hiv-and-aids-timeline
3. Thomas E. The New Untouchables. 1985, September 23. Accessed May 2019. http://content.time.com/time/magazine/article/0,9171,959944,00.html#ixzz1ODE14wsi
4. U.S. FDA. Practice Hospital Bed Safety. 2013, February 11. Accessed June 2019. https://www.fda.gov/consumers/consumer-updates/practice-hospital-bed-safety
5. Donskey CJ. Does Improving Surface Cleaning and Disinfection Reduce Health Care-Associated Infections? *American Journal of Infection Control* 2013. 41(5):S12–S19.
6. Suwantarat N, LA Supple, JL Cadnum, T Sankar, and CJ Donskey. Quantitative Assessment of Interactions between Hospitalized Patients and Portable Medical Equipment and Other Fomites. *American Journal of Infection Control* 2017. 45(11):1276–1278.
7. Twentyman J. Hacking Medical Devices Is the Next Big Security Concern. *Financial Times*. 2017, November 8. Accessed August 2019. https://www.ft.com/content/75912040-98ad-11e7-8c5c-c8d8fa6961bb
8. Waqas. How a Coffee Machine Infected Factory Computers with Ransomware. Hackread.com 2017, July 28. Accessed July 2019. https://www.hackread.com/how-a-coffee-machine-infected-factory-computers-with-ransomware/
9. Brewster T. How to Hack Someone Off a Segway Scooter in 20 Seconds. *Forbes*. 2017, July 19. Accessed July 2019. https://www.forbes.com/sites/thomasbrewster/2017/07/19/segway-hoverboard-hacked-in-20-seconds/#1efa6d2f113f
10. Astor M. Your Roomba May be Mapping Your Home, Collecting Data that Could Be Shared. *New York Times*.2017, July 25. Accessed July 2019. https://www.nytimes.com/2017/07/25/technology/roomba-irobot-data-privacy.html?mtrref=www.google.co.uk&mtrref=www.nytimes.com&gwh=0DDB21FCA8B9215A63DFBFE41917210F&gwt=pay
11. Perakslis E. Cyber Security Modeled as Infection Prevention and Control in the Healthcare Delivery Setting. *BMJ Blog*. 2017, May 16.
12. Ponemon Institute. 2015 State of the Endpoint Report: User-Centric Risk. 2015, January. Accessed July 2019. https://www.ponemon.org/local/upload/file/2015%20State%20of%20Endpoint%20Risk%20FINAL.pdf

5

Pulse Oximetry in Anesthesia—The "Perfect" Medical Technology Use Case

Although often thought of as futuristic, my first digital health project began in 1986. At the time, I was a sophomore college student and Biomedical Engineering intern and my second-year project was to assist with the implementation of the first pulse oximeters. The program provided clear and significant benefits to patients, clinicians, and the hospital. I have seldom seen this type of clear and uniform value across the care continuum since then.

Commonplace now, pulse oximetry was first commercialized in the 1980s and provided a noninvasive, real-time measurement of oxygen saturation, the fraction of oxygen-saturated hemoglobin relative to the total hemoglobin in blood.[1] At the time, the best practice was the measurement of arterial blood gas via an arterial blood draw/catheter and stat analysis in the hospital lab. Although the arterial blood gas analysis provided more information (pH, partial pressures, carbonates, total hemoglobin, etc.), executing the test was challenging. It was hoped that these new machines would offer clear benefits to patients, clinicians, and healthcare institutions. Our job was to test these things in our real-life setting.

Risks of anesthesia

According to the Anesthesia Quality Institute's National Anesthesia Clinical Outcomes Registry (NACOR) of anesthesia cases in all settings, from hospitals to freestanding clinics, there were more than 5.9 million non-Operating Room (OR) anesthesia cases and 12.4 million OR cases from 2010 through 2014, with the trend of non-OR cases increasing from 28% to 34% during this period of time.[2] The process of anesthesia is actually far more complex than many imagine. According to Bill Perkins at the Mayo College of Medicine in Rochester, Minnesota, Oliver Wendell Holmes coined the term "anesthesia" in 1846 to describe drug-induced insensibility to sensation (particularly

Digital Health. Eric D. Perakslis and Martin Stanley, Oxford University Press (2021). © Oxford University Press.
DOI: 10.1093/oso/9780197503133.003.0005

pain), shortly after the first publicized demonstration of inhaled ether rendered a patient unresponsive during a surgical procedure.[3]

In general, there are three major classes of anesthesia: local, regional, and general. Local and regional anesthetics pharmacologically block nerve transmission to pain centers in the central nervous system via obstruction of the movement of nerve impulses near the site of injection, but there are no changes in awareness and sense perception in other areas. In contrast, general anesthetics induce a different sort of anesthetic state, one of general insensibility to pain. The patient loses awareness yet his vital physiologic functions, such as breathing and maintenance of blood pressure, continue to function. Believe it or not, despite more than 150 years of use, far less is known about the mechanism of action of general anesthetics compared to local anesthetic agents such as Novocain. This lack of knowledge makes it difficult to predict in advance which patients may be more likely to experience side effects. The implications of this can be significant when all other known risk factors, such as age, severity of illness etc., are not present.

One of the more common expressions used to describe general anesthesia is "putting patients to sleep" (a phrase that is used for a very different context in veterinary medicine). It is more accurate, however, to think of general anesthesia as a drug-induced coma, given that brain activity (as measured by electroencephalogram, or EEG) dips down to levels akin to brain-stem death.[4] This coma-like state necessitates careful monitoring of breathing, body temperature, ECG, and blood oxygenation, as well as the delicate balancing of "hypnotic agents, inhalational agents, opioids, muscle relaxants, sedatives, and cardiovascular drugs that are used."

Coincidentally, the American Society of Anesthesiologists published the *Standards for Basic Anesthetic Monitoring* in October 1986, which coincided with the time frame of our pulse oximetry pilots. Most recently revised in 2015, the standards specify two major requirements: (1) Qualified anesthesia personnel shall be present in the room throughout the conduct of all general anesthetics, regional anesthetics, and monitored anesthesia care; (2) During all anesthetics, the patient's oxygenation, ventilation, circulation, and temperature shall be continually evaluated.[5] Looking more closely at the requirements for oxygenation, ventilation, and circulation, the standard explicitly states that adequate oxygen concentration in the inspired gas and the blood during all anesthetics must be ensured. Appropriate methods include specific measurements for inspired gas. Specifically, during every administration of general anesthesia using an anesthesia machine, the concentration of oxygen in the patient breathing system shall be measured by an oxygen analyzer with a low-oxygen concentration limit alarm in use. The second element is blood oxygenation wherein, during all anesthetics, a quantitative method of assessing oxygenation such as pulse oximetry shall be employed. When the pulse oximeter is utilized, the variable pitch pulse tone and the low threshold alarm shall be audible to the anesthesiologist or the anesthesia care team personnel. Of course, the pulse oximetry requirement did not yet exist in 1986, because blood gases were the standard of care at that time. These standards have evolved over time in an effort to minimize the risks of anesthesia, but risks remain. According to the American Society of Anesthesiologists,

> Surgery and anesthesia are safer today than ever before, thanks to continuing advances in science. But this doesn't mean there is zero risk. In fact, surgery and anesthesia are inherently dangerous, and as with any medication or procedure, there is always the chance that something can go wrong. Certain patients are more likely to experience problems or complications and possibly even death than others because of their age, medical conditions or the type of surgery they're having. If you're planning to have surgery, there are ways to lower your risk, including meeting with your physician anesthesiologist.[6]

More specifically, allergies to the anesthetic drugs, other adverse drug events, heart disease, high blood pressure, kidney problems, lung conditions, obesity, and obstructive sleep apnea are all factors that increase the risks of general anesthesia. These risk factors increase the probability of adverse events such as postoperative delirium and/or cognitive dysfunction, malignant hyperthermia, a serious, potentially deadly reaction to anesthesia that can occur during surgery, causing a quick fever and muscle contractions and breathing problems before or after surgery.

Blood gas monitoring yesterday and today

The gold standard for assessing respiratory status is the arterial blood gas analysis (ABG). Blood samples are taken either via single arterial puncture or an arterial catheter. Relative contraindications include bleeding diathesis or disturbance of clotting factors. According to DC Flenley, who published a detailed overview of arterial puncture in the *British Medical Journal* in 1980, "drawing blood from an artery requires expertise and skill and can be painful for the patient. It is also a time-consuming process that carries a certain risk for infection and damage of tissue, nerves, and vessels.[7] The purpose of ABG analysis has traditionally been to measure blood acidity, pH, and the levels of oxygen (O_2) and carbon dioxide (CO_2) in the blood as a way to watch acute and chronic respiratory failure, transport, cardiopulmonary resuscitation, patient-controlled analgesia, and procedural sedation. Attempts at modernizing and automating blood gas analysis date back to the 1950s when the first three-function blood gas analyzer, an instrument capable of measuring pH, the partial pressure of oxygen (pO_2), and the partial pressure of carbon dioxide (pCO_2) was developed in 1959 by John W. Severinghaus MD, an anesthesiologist and innovator, and Freeman A. Bradley, his laboratory technician.[8] Interestingly, one of the primary drivers for arterial blood gas measurement was the unmet needs of polio patients requiring artificial ventilation during the epidemics of the early 1950s.

On the surface, arterial blood gas analysis was fairly common and somewhat automated by the mid-1980s. An anesthesiologist or nurse anesthetist would start an arterial line as part of the initiation of anesthesia and could pull blood samples as needed at any time during sedation as long as the arterial catheter remained available, properly in place, and unobstructed. However, inserting arterial lines is difficult and painful enough that it does not happen to every patient undergoing general anesthesia. One unmet need was the instance of rare side effects for otherwise healthy patients. I remember one such example vividly. The planned procedure was a simple scope to clean up and repair a knee injury in a very healthy teenage female athlete. This young lady had an allergic reaction to one of the anesthetic agents, ketamine, and was very quickly in danger. I vividly remember helping to restrain and protect the unconscious patient while she convulsed wildly on the table. The anesthesiologist, one hand bracing the patient's chin, to keep the ventilation apparatus in place, and the other hand working calmly across the range of medical gas vaporizers until the patient settled down and was sedated comfortably. The young lady recovered fully and was back in a few weeks to have her knee procedure successfully and without incident. This taught me how quickly the quiet and almost dull rhythm of the operating room can turn to what would appear to be chaos to an unfamiliar observer. It also taught me the difficulty of arterial puncture during an emergency. An arterial line had not been started on this patient due to her lack of risk factors, and it was clearly not possible to do so during the acute episode of her drug reaction.

The pulse oximeter validation project was a study where we ran both technologies in parallel. We installed pulse oximeters onto the anesthesia stations in several of the operating suites and the anesthesiologists were trained by the device manufacturer. The devices were tested head-to-head via comparison with arterial blood gas draws. Thirty years later, I still have vivid memories of assisting during the insertions of arterial catheters, which was difficult and painful. Drawing arterial blood is complex, because arteries can be difficult to palpate and catheterize. It was clearly quite painful for awake patients and difficult for all involved. Further, the sample of blood had to be properly handled and the test run in less than 30 minutes due to rapid sample degradation. The sample was immediately iced and quickly transported to the lab. We then waited for the results to be conveyed by phone back to the operating room (OR). The process was long, cumbersome, and scaled poorly across a dozen simultaneously active operating suites. This was the process we hoped to replace.

A pulse oximeter is able to noninvasively measure the amount of oxygen-saturated hemoglobin (oxyhemoglobin) in a patient's arterial blood. Going back to the history provided by Witt, the science behind this amazing feat was mostly understood by 1852 when German physicist August Beer proved that the amount of light transmitted through a solution varies based on the concentration of solute. The next contributing discovery was in 1939 when a German physician, Karl Matthes, showed that oxyhemoglobin could be measured in the ear via utilization of two different wavelengths of light: red and infrared. Infrared is absorbed more by oxygenated hemoglobin and red more by deoxygenated hemoglobin. The term "oximeter" was coined by Glenn Milliken when he applied the capability to the measurement of oxygen saturation in pilots during World War II. Additional increments moved the technology forward until the last major breakthrough was made by a Japanese electrical engineer, Takuo Aoyagi, who figured out that the difference in light absorption during a pulsation and between pulsations, represented only arterial flow and represented the difference between peak saturation and baseline. This eliminated the need for pneumatic pressure, which previously had been required to measure baseline in the absence of blood. This also enabled the development of devices that could measure pulse oximetry without the need for arterial or venous catheters. Of course, these devices are not flawless. In particular, situations such as carbon monoxide poisoning can cause the presence of molecules that have similar absorption to oxyhemoglobin and can confound readings.

Benefit-risk assessment

The first pulse oximeters, Nellcor's in our case, replaced this painful invasive approach with a simple, soft, clothes pin-like clip placed over a finger.[9] In addition to the clinical benefits, in 1986 dollars, for every anesthesia station in the OR and/or Labor and Delivery ward that we installed and qualified, each anesthesiologist saved approximately $3,000 in liability insurance.

Analysis of the benefits and risks of this transformation demonstrates extremely significant clinical and financial benefits obtained while reducing the overall risk of procedures to a very low level. A complex, painful, episodic, and manually intensive procedure was replaced with a noninvasive, painless, real-time, digital measurement. Although less information-rich than the antecedent, the pulse oximeter proved to be more useful long term, as the real-time ability allowed anesthetists to follow trends over time that could indicate oxygen desaturation or other complications instantly. If more detailed analysis was needed at any time, a blood gas could still be drawn and measured. Truly a win-win-win, the benefits for patients, providers, and the healthcare institution were clear and striking.

In the 30 years since this effort, I have seldom seen such a clear-cut benefit-risk determination. One of the most lasting impressions from my time with these studies was running the arterial blood samples in a Styrofoam cup full of ice down several floors to the pathology lab and running up again to wait near the phone in the operating suite to hear the results. Sometimes, it was mundane. Other times, it was tense or clearly urgent. In all cases, the primary impression I retain is that the process started at the bedside with the patient. A world of rapidly evolving science terms such as "bench-to-bedside" are used to discuss the translation of technological advancement to direct benefits for patients. Sometimes that works. In my experience it is innovation that starts at the bedside that has a higher chance of success, impact, and value.

References

1. Witt C. Vital Signs Are Vital: The History of Pulse Oximetry. *ACP Hospitalist*. 2014, May. Accessed September 2019 https://acphospitalist.org/archives/2014/05/newman.htm
2. American Society of Anesthesiologists. More Americans Undergo Anesthesia Outside of the O.R. https://www.asahq.org/about-asa/newsroom/news-releases/2016/10/more-americans-undergo-procedures-involving-anesthesia-outside-or
3. Perkins B. How Does Anesthesia Work? *Scientific American*. 2005, February 7. Accessed August 2019. https://www.scientificamerican.com/article/how-does-anesthesia-work/
4. Harmon K. The Body Under General Anesthesia Tracks Closer to Coma than Sleep. *Scientific American*. 2010, December 29. Accessed August 2019. https://www.scientificamerican.com/article/general-anesthesia-coma/
5. AHRQ, American Society of Anesthesiologists. Standards for Basic Anesthetic Monitoring. 1986, October 21. Accessed August 2019.

6. American Society of Anesthesiologists. When Seconds Count. Anesthesia 101. Anesthesia Risks. Accessed August 2019. https://www.asahq.org/whensecondscount/anesthesia-101/anesthesia-risks/

7. Flenley DC. Procedures in Practice: Arterial Puncture. *BMJ*. 1980, July 12. 281(6233), 128–131.

8. Severinghaus JW. The Invention and Development of Blood Gas Analysis Apparatus. *Anesthesiology 7* 2002. 97, 253–256.

9. Wood Library Museum. Nellcor Pulse Oximeter. Record. WLM ID: akfr. Accessed August 2019. https://www.woodlibrarymuseum.org/museum/item/531/nellcor-pulse-oximeter

6

The Technology of Biotechnology and Big Data in Medicine Development

Switching gears from the direct patient-care setting, this chapter looks at technology evolution in biomedical product development. The relationships between medicine, drug, device, and diagnostic development can be a bit confusing. Stated simply, in the United States, the Food and Drug Administration (FDA) regulates the tools that health care uses but not the practice of health care. In fact, the two exist in barely overlapping ways, which presents challenges and opportunities, because the lessons learned within each do not necessarily flow seamlessly toward the other.

The cures factory

During the middle and late 1990s, as the Internet and Windows operating systems started to make computers accessible and necessary for professional and home use, the biotechnology field was rapidly incorporating these new capabilities. Prior to this era, drug discovery had been primarily low-tech. The process of finding new medicines revolved around in vivo (taking part in living organisms) pharmacology studies, most often in rats and mice. There was an extensive and growing set of animal models available that mimicked specific disease conditions and scientists would design and synthesize molecules to be tested in these models for biological activity. Although low-tech from the standpoint of computing power, the process itself was supported by a significant amount of highly specialized technology. The identity and purity of complex organic molecules was determined, tracked, and optimized via advanced analytical chemistry machinery at a low level of throughput. The optimization of chemical and biological hypothesis led to the need for rendering extremely similar versions of molecules in an iterative process to optimize biological activity and minimize any potential toxicities that could eventually translate into side effects of the new drug.

In the late 1990s, Chris Lipinski and others published a paper that drove a computational revolution in drug discovery. The paper, "Experimental and

Digital Health. Eric D. Perakslis and Martin Stanley, Oxford University Press (2021). © Oxford University Press.
DOI: 10.1093/oso/9780197503133.003.0006

Computational Approaches to Estimate Solubility and Permeability in Drug Discovery and Development Settings," provided the first easily programmable rubric for a small set of attributes that determines whether a molecule is "drug-like."[1] The "Lipinski Rule of 5," as it would come to be known stated simply that a molecule was not "drug-like," specifically would have poor biological absorption and permeation, if the molecule had more than 5 H-bond donors, 10 H-bond acceptors, the molecular weight (MWT) were greater than 500, and the calculated Log P (CLogP) were greater than 5. This simple model transformed drug hunting by establishing a set of criteria perfectly suited to drive computation on a massive scale.

Specifically, if you take all the known elements from the periodic table and all the associated known properties, currently 118 at the time of this writing, you can easily write computer algorithms to combinatorialize, develop every possible combination, resulting in a list of every molecule that could possibly be synthesized. You can then cull the list down by excluding radioactive and known poisonous elements, given that these would probably not be the best candidates as medications. The Lipinski Rule of 5 appeared at the perfect point in time to refine this combinatorial process even further. The result of this advance was a surge in investment in small biotechnology companies striving to optimize the opportunity this approach presented.

In 1996, just a year before the Lipinski paper, I started my first "real" job in biotech at a small company named ArQule located in Medford, Massachusetts just a few miles down the road from my first hospital job a decade earlier. The original business strategy of ArQule was to exploit the automation of combinatorial chemistry at scale by manufacturing large libraries of molecules that would be licensed to pharmaceutical, biotechnology, and agrichemical companies to screen for candidate molecules for their research and development (R&D) programs. Each year between 100,000 and 200,000 molecules were synthesized in smaller batches that we called libraries. Libraries averaged 5,000–10,000 molecules each and represented a distinct chemistry that was represented by a unique Markush structure, a representation of chemical structure used to indicate a group of related chemical compounds, which are commonly used in chemistry texts and in patent claims. We would make multiple copies of these libraries and ship them in 96-well microtiter plates to our many collaborators. This meant that partners understood the basic chemistry of the compounds within a library but not the exact structures of each molecule in a library, and they had no idea of what molecule was within any given well on the microtiter plates. The model was such that our partners would "screen" the molecules in their bioassays and report the physical location of any "hits," that is, highly active molecules as determined by their assays.

The nature of this type of drug discovery process optimizes the structure-activity relationship (SAR) of candidate molecules. Simply put, SAR is the relationship between the chemical structure and the biological activity of a molecule. In drug discovery, once a hit is identified, it often is optimized via the synthesis of new molecules, each with a small but distinct chemical difference. These molecules are then screened in the bioassay to see whether the small changes make the molecule more or less active. The process continues until an optimal candidate molecule is achieved. Combinatorial chemistry and high-throughput bioassays were capable of mass automation in a way that almost replaced the previous model of SAR development, which was based solely upon the intuition of biologists and chemists.[2] While we were building the chemical synthesis potential, biopharmaceutical companies were building the massive compound management and bioassay screening capabilities, often highly robotic, to hunt down and identify the most promising candidate molecules.

The first "dirty" data

Against this backdrop of drug discovery automation, the human genome project was in full swing and rapidly approaching completion.[3] The hope of the day was that all this technology would enable a simple, statistical approach to drug hunting. The human genome project would illuminate the basic mechanisms of disease. These mechanisms could then be targeted by highly specific and fully automated bioassays that would be fed via a constant supply of hundreds of thousands of unique molecules from companies such as ArQule.[4] The safety of candidate molecules would be similarly optimized via highly automated toxicology screens that would quickly and effectively remove "bad" molecules from consideration. The overall result would be massive increases in the number of new drugs discovered. In practice it did not work out this way for reasons that are essential to understanding the landscape today, in which technologies such as machine learning, artificial intelligence, and miniaturized biosensors are being touted, and fetishized, as imminent solutions for the complexity of health care and human disease.

Fast forward to 1999, when I am now employed at a pharmaceutical research division of Johnson & Johnson (J&J) and am witnessing the bioassay side of the process. Having been recruited to J&J from ArQule to develop chemo-informatic solutions, I quickly begin to see the challenges in implementing highly automated drug discovery. I also hear the expression "dirty data" for the first time. One of the unavoidable differences between robots synthesizing thousands of molecules at scale and a single chemist creating one molecule at a time is purity. The automated process at ArQule was designed to average 85% purity of each molecule compared to chemists working one molecule at a time who average better than 99%. These differences quickly led to reduced trust in the products of automation. The most frequent case was when a highly active well in a microtiter plate was not confirmed when the expected molecule that well contained was synthesized and tested independently. This cast doubt upon the entire process, given that the root cause(s) were seldom obvious. Was the lack of confirmation due to poor-quality assay? Was it because the well was only 85% pure and the actual bioactivity was due to the impurity or impurities within the remaining 15%? These questions were often difficult to answer and would stall progress in drug hunting programs. Eventually, the accusation of "dirty data" would arise, wherein the initial excitement over hits on these automated platforms was quickly replaced, first with disappointment and next with skepticism. The latter being significantly exacerbated by the fact that many drug discovery scientists viewed these technologies as genuine threats to their livelihood as they increasingly feared being replaced by automation. From an economic perspective, those fears were not unfounded. Using a few basic assumptions of the time, a productive organic chemist could synthesize 100–200 highly pure molecules per year depending on the complexity of the required chemistry, and a biologist could screen a few thousand molecules a year for biological activity. Assuming a fully loaded full-time equivalent (FTE) salary plus all benefits, cost of roughly $250,000 per year in 1999 dollars this roughly works out to a cost of a little more than $1,000/molecule for synthesis and a few hundred dollars per molecule for bioassay screening. By comparison, automated high-throughput screening platforms averaged $7–$8 per well screened and translated to a cost benefit of 10X–20X. Although full automation was tempting it was not a significant motivation. The concept was that the machines would do the heavy lifting for primary screening and the humans would optimize the resulting leads. More often than not, this led to the reproducibility issues previously described and mistrust of the dirty data. These lines of thinking are not unalike what we see today with artificial intelligence in health care. Will AI make pathologists and radiologists obsolete? Is it safe to trust algorithms in clinical medicine? Who is liable, etc.?

According to Wikipedia, dirty data are inaccurate, incomplete, or inconsistent data, especially in a computer system or database.[5] This is a great starting point. If we look at high-throughput screening data more closely, there are many elements involved. First, there is the relative purity and impurity of the compound in the well. What exactly is causing positive bioactivity of a well containing 85% expected compound and 15% impurity or impurities? Is it the target compound? Is it one of the impurities? Is it a combination of the impurities? Is it a combination of one of the impurities and the expected primary compound? In addition to uncertainties about the chemical composition of the screened molecule, the bioassays themselves also had known and unknown rates of accompanying error. Having to disaggregate the many possibilities of this situation is complex. Given that systems were producing this occurrence hundreds of times per day, it is understandable why these approaches eventually were mostly abandoned by the mid-2000s.

But was the data dirty based upon the above definition? Probably, yes, in that the bioassay was producing a single numerical result on every well despite the myriad of mitigating factors that varied by well. This is especially true when the group studying the data are the exact people who had traditionally done these tasks much more slowly and painstakingly. It was self-assuring to conclude that automation results in dirty data while humans produce far more valuable "clean" data. This oft-repeated narrative catches on quickly whenever the machines are "threatening" human jobs, but it is not always true. Indeed, much of the auto industry now uses welding and assembly robots, which perform far more precisely than individual humans ever did. The conundrum is actually more about whether science can be automated as effectively as manufacturing.

Once established, the term dirty data has been exploited, overused, and poorly used. For example, patient-reported outcome (PRO) data from clinical trials has frequently been referred to as "dirty," given that it can be inaccurate and inconsistent.[6,7] There are many reasons for this, such as patient bias, lack of scientific understanding, and a host of psychological factors that may influence what a patient decides to report on a given PRO instrument. But do those things actually make the data dirty if the patient really believes them to be true? This lack of precision is critically important in understanding how humans, technology, media, and truth intersect in the current day. When does data become so dirty that it is actually fake? And what is truth? How do we examine data without confirmation bias? How do we deal with the many other factors, virtuous and not, that drive scientific and public opinion? We will dive into these topics much more deeply in the upcoming chapters and sections on medical misinformation, disinformation, and malinformation.

Technology in clinical trials

Technology in clinical trials has changed very little over the last few decades from the standpoint of what is measured clinically, how it is measured, and how it is reported. For patients, researchers, or clinicians, the most authoritative source for metrics on clinical trials, as well as information on individual trials, is clinicaltrials.gov.[8] This site, maintained by the National Library of Medicine (NLM) at the National Institutes of Health (NIH), has been in operation since February 2000 and is the authoritative source for data on medical studies on human volunteers. The site is a great example of not letting the perfect be the enemy of the good. Although it receives its fair share of criticism over imperfections, the site serves its intended purpose and is by far the most authoritative source for clinical trials data. Indeed, most significant statistics to reference originate from this source. As of October 2, 2019, there were 318,280 trials registered at clinicaltrials. gov. Of this number, 79% were interventional and 21% were observational. Of the interventional studies, 141,866 were drug or biologic studies, 80,578 were behavioral or other, 26,490 were surgical procedures, and 32,012 were device studies. Of the 318,280 trials registered, only 39,209 studies (roughly 12%) contained posted results. One of the major criticisms of clinicaltrials.gov is that the data is inconsistent and incomplete, but as with many systems, incomplete data usually indicates issues with usage versus the system itself. The data in clinicaltrials.gov is incomplete simply because the individuals who register trials into the system seldom complete their submission once a trial has completed, especially if the trial failed. A study of clinical trials that posted final results and those that did not published in the *New England Journal of Medicine* in 2015, found that timely reporting was independently associated with factors such as FDA oversight, a later trial phase, and industry funding.[9]

The three main components of clinical trial design are the experimental design, the statistical design, and the analysis plan. The experimental plan includes the statement of the problem, the objective of the study, the choice of response variable, the selection of factors to be varied, and the choice of levels of these factors (fixed, random, quantitative, or qualitative). The statistical design includes the sample size, the method of randomization, the mathematical models to be utilized, the hypothesis, and blinding procedure. The analysis plan covers things such as data collection and processing, computation of test statistics, preparation of graphics and tables, and the interpretation of results.[10] Expanding upon some of the key terms, randomization is the process of assigning patients to different groups based entirely upon chance and is intended to prevent bias. Blinding is the process used to ensure people involved in the clinical trial do not know which patients are assigned to which group. It also prevents bias. Bias is defined as any tendency that prevents unprejudiced consideration of a question.[11]

Many types of bias can occur at any phase in clinical trials, and great care must be taken at every stage to eliminate all possible manifestations; otherwise, the basic comparisons within a study can be flawed or invalid. It is important to note that even with proper randomization and blinding, many other potential sources of bias exist, such as conflicts of interest, patients being lost to follow-up (dropping out of the trial), and numerous others. Indeed, one review of sources of bias and bias prevalence in clinical studies in the *American Journal of Epidemiology* determined that adequate randomization, blinding, and follow-up may be important in bias control, but the influence of the various components in individual trials cannot be predicted.[12]

The role of clinical data management (CDM) is to ensure high-quality, reliable, and regulatorily compliant data from clinical trials. It is essentially the full documentation from study design through regulatory filing, if applicable, all the way through long-term records management. There are many distinct documents, metadata and artifacts including case report forms (CRF) that document each individual patient interaction, clinical databases, statistical databases, protocol documentation, training materials, safety and protocol deviation, exception reporting, and many other documents. Interestingly, CDM is considered a competitive space, given that companies often are developing similar drugs at the same time. Being able to document a trial properly and submit the findings more quickly can be a competitive advantage. For these reasons and due to the inherent complexity of the process, there has historically been an active and competitive software market. Over the years, products such as ORACLE CLINICAL, CLINTRIAL, MACRO, RAVE, and *e*Clinical Suite have competed for dominance and market share.[13] Overall, this has been seen as a good thing from the standpoint of compliance, because regulatory rigor can usually be more easily confirmed when fewer, more highly standardized systems are employed, compared to decades ago when each biopharma company had a proprietary system that could take a regulator weeks or months to understand during an audit.

The other advantage of a more consolidated software market relates to documentation of regulatory compliance. In biomedical product development, computer systems must be "validated" to ensure proper traceability, accountability, and data integrity. This process is often referred to as (GXP) compliance.[14] As stated earlier, GLP refers to Good Laboratory Practices and GCP refers to Good Clinical Practices. The term GXP is used for computer systems, because there is only one validation standard that is applicable to all computer systems regardless of whether they are supporting laboratory, clinical, or manufacturing processes. The expense and complexity of managing GXP compliance across a drug development portfolio of dozens of compounds has been a significant driver in consolidation of the clinical trial management software market, because implementations can vary very little from company to company. Software-as-a-Service (SaaS) implementations, in which the software is actually hosted by the software vendor, further diminish complexity as the underlying hosting infrastructure also is standardized.[15]

Regulatory requirements

From the standpoint of data, the purpose of clinical trial data is inclusion in a regulatory filing for marketing authorization. This is the process of reviewing and assessing evidence to determine: whether the drug is safe and effective in its proposed use(s); whether the benefits of the drug outweigh the risks; whether the drug's proposed labeling (package insert) is appropriate and contains everything it should; and whether the methods used in manufacturing the drug and the controls used to maintain the drug's quality are adequate to preserve the drug's identity, strength, quality, and purity.[16] The flow of data from each clinical interaction, into the EHRs of clinical sites, through the clinical trials systems, and into New Drug Application filings (in the United States) is often complex due to the need for double entry and other forms of redundancy.

One way to understand this chain of data is starting with a single patient interaction. The clinical trial protocol lists the patient entry criteria. Clinical sites are contracted, directly by the product sponsor or, more typically, subcontracted through clinical research organizations (CROs). Sites are selected based on the presence of lead clinicians, called site primary investigators (PIs), who have access to large populations of the intended patients via their clinical and research practices. Once a site is selected it must be initiated and authorized by a rigorous set of processes including prestudy qualification and qualification visits. The purpose of these processes is to ensure that adequate staffing, policies, and procedures exist to execute the clinical trial in a fully safe and compliant manner. The documentation required for the initiation of a single site is extensive. The complexity grows rapidly, because most large trials involve many sites where the resulting data must be merged seamlessly into databases, documents, and regulatory filings.

Getting back to that single patient, once enrolled in the study, each clinical encounter must be fully documented. The basic data-capture mechanism is the case report form (CRF). The International Conference on Harmonization Guidelines for Good Clinical Practice define the CRF as: A printed, optical, or electronic document designed to record all of the protocol-required information to be reported to the sponsor on each trial subject.[17] The CRF fills the purpose of documenting the clinical interaction for the clinical trial but not for the purposes of clinical care within the site, which is typically managed via the site EHR. This most often leads to data reentry, which is not only extra work, but also often error-prone and unaligned from the standpoint of data collected, given that the CRF and EHR contain different data elements for different purposes. This introduces error and adds expense, complexity, and compliance risk to the trial. In a more ideal world, clinical interactions would be captured in a single manner that was adequate for research and patient care.

Once a trial is completed and the final applications have been negotiated, submitted, reviewed, and approved by regulatory authorities, the penultimate data artifact is the label. The content and management requirements for medical-product labels are extremely detailed and complex. For example, in the United States, drug labels are codified in 21CFR201.56.[18] In lieu of an attempt to summarize the extensive content required, I suggest the reader take a close look at this document, because there is simply no better way to obtain an understanding of the extent and complexity of product labeling regulation. Suffice it to say that the regulations are long, detailed, and extremely difficult to understand or to comply with without significant international infrastructure, and this is as it should be given the ultimate importance of product labeling.

Clinical trial knowledge management

Intentional proactive knowledge management strategies are one of the most overlooked aspects of clinical data management and, therefore, one of the greatest opportunities it offers. If you follow the regulatory lifecycle of clinical data, after the product is licensed and launched into the market, the focus becomes safety monitoring, line extensions, and lifecycle management. The safety monitoring and line extension parts may go hand-in-hand and can be quite active with new products, especially during the first few years, because clinicians and researchers likely will be actively testing the products in new populations over time. Some of this is planned well in advance, even before the phase III clinical trial, such as when it had been decided to omit certain populations for safety reasons. Hence, studies in women of childbearing age, children, specific ethnic groups, patient groups that have a preexisting condition, etc., all are examples of populations that may have been omitted from registry trials but that may offer the first opportunities for line extensions. Other activities include experimentation in new indications (diseases), filings in other countries, and following and interpreting safety data that comes in on a daily basis.

All of these activities result in novel content being delivered to the drug sponsor, which, if more easily leveraged, could yield significant insight beyond the sum of the parts. This seldom happens, because the data often is returned in an ad-hoc fashion to different parts of the organization. Clinical trial results go to the therapeutic area strategy team and clinical operations. Safety data go to the pharmacovigilance (drug safety) group and to the regulatory affairs group, both of which must work together to interpret and report safety data and recommendations to the appropriate regulatory authorities. The master database for each product is usually the labeling system, which must keep track of every label element, on each product, in every language.

Outside of the labeling database, much of the data that is aggregated into sponsors' systems as part of lifecycle management remains fragmented. The results are architectures that are functional and domain driven. For example, all the scientific data from clinical trials is often in SAS databases, a statistical software suite developed by SAS Institute for advanced analytics, multivariate analysis, business intelligence, criminal investigation, data management, and predictive analytics. The operational elements are likely in a Clinical Trial Management System (CTMS). The regulatory filings are within regulatory operations (Reg Ops) databases, the protocol and Standard Operating Procedures (SOPs) are in a document store, etc. Although it would be logical to assume that companies would be highly incentivized to bring this data together for educational purposes, data protection, and records management, this is often not the case. First and foremost, data consolidation efforts can be quite lengthy and expensive if knowledge management was not designed into the data architecture from the beginning. This often results in any further data consolidation being considered solely according to a cost-benefit analysis of the value of anything new being learned from the investment.

Trials in devices

There are significant differences in the approach of clinical trials for medical devices as opposed to drugs. First, the definition of medical device is less clear than that of therapeutics agents. According to the U.S. FDA, a device is, "an instrument, apparatus, implement, machine, contrivance, implant, in vitro reagent, or other similar or related article, including a component part, or accessory which is:

1. *recognized in the official National Formulary, or the United States Pharmacopoeia, or any supplement to them,*
2. *intended for use in the diagnosis of disease or other conditions, or in the cure, mitigation, treatment, or prevention of disease, in man or other animals, or*
3. *intended to affect the structure or any function of the body of man or other animals, and which does not achieve its primary intended purposes through chemical action within or on the body of man or other animals and*

which does not achieve its primary intended purposes through chemical action within or on the body of man or other animals and which is not dependent upon being metabolized for the achievement of its primary intended purposes. The term 'device' does not include software functions excluded pursuant to section 520(o)."[19]

As straightforward as these definitions appear, the rapidly evolving field of digital health blurs these classifications. For example, many consumer-grade wearable technologies now gather data that had previously only been provided by medical devices, such as electrocardiogram data. To date, the approach of the FDA is to determine which classifications specific devices belong to and to regulate those that are traditional medical devices and to not regulate those that are not. There are valid concerns that this approach will be gamed by predatory actors that will continue to push medical advantages of devices that are not properly regulated.

The clinical trials process for medical devices is quite different than the trial process for drugs; trials for devices tend to be smaller, are difficult or impossible to randomize or blind, may depend heavily on the skill of the user (e.g., in the case of surgical devices), are likely to involve modifications to the devices during the trial, and have highly diverse endpoints.[20] From a process perspective, there are essentially three types of studies: exploratory or feasibility studies for proof of concept, pivotal studies to demonstrate safety and efficacy, and postmarketing studies to better understand the utility and long-term safety of the device.[21]

Despite the many differences in scope, scale, and purpose, the technologies employed to manage medical device trials are not significantly different than those used in drug trials. CTMS, document management, and

GxP validation and label management are all fairly analogous and the data-system approaches at a large medical device sponsor would have a great deal in common with those at a large biopharmaceutical sponsor. Small innovator companies with only one or two low-risk products, however, are very different. The infrastructure at those companies resembles a consumer electronics shop.

Real world evidence, remote trials, and synthetic patients

By far, some of the most interesting work and opportunity in clinical trial technologies is in paradigm-shifting trial operating models. It is important to note that these models have received a significant increase in focus due to the COVID-19 pandemic, which had initially resulted in many trial stoppages due to infection control and patient safety concerns, as well as the closure of many traditional clinical research sites during the pandemic.

We will consider three such models: Remote trials will be defined as trials that occur outside of typical clinical sites; virtual trials will refer to retrospective or prospective *in silico* study of clinical hypothesis in data sets, and real-world evidence will refer to data collected in the course of normal medical practice, which could include EHR data, medical claims data, or similarly aggregated content.

Statistics show that clinical trial participation is linked to the geography of the trial location.[22] Most patients do not live close to a major academic center where clinical trials are being performed, and the burden of travel makes participation prohibitive for many patients. The ideal situation would bring clinical trials to patients wherever they are, but this is extremely complex, given that the infrastructure, compliance, personnel, and many other human and technology systems are prohibitively expensive and complex.[23] Several excellent attempts to address these challenges have been made. For more than a decade, companies such as MYTRUS have built digital health technologies to enable patients to participate remotely via electronic data capture and local medical management. This is truly a place where modern mobile technologies should shine, but, to date, this has not happened due to market dynamics. In recent years, these types of companies have been gobbled up via acquisition, primarily by the large clinical trial CROs. In most cases to date, the technologies have been validated and repurposed toward traditional clinical research models. In some ways, this should be viewed as confirmation that remote trials hold great potential for patients and as an argument for the disruption of the current CRO industrial complex.

Real-world evidence (RWE) is defined by the U.S. FDA as clinical evidence regarding the usage and potential benefits or risks of a medical product derived from analysis of real-world data (RWD). RWE can be generated by different study designs or analyses, including but not limited to, randomized trials, including large simple trials, pragmatic trials, and observational studies (prospective and/or retrospective).[24] RWD are defined as data relating to patient health status and/or the delivery of health care routinely collected from a variety of sources, such as,

- Electronic health records (EHRs)
- Claims and billing activities
- Product and disease registries
- Patient-generated data including in-home-use settings
- Data gathered from other sources that can inform on health status, such as mobile devices.

For regulatory purposes, RWE is being used for the monitoring of postmarket safety, to support coverage decisions, for use in clinical decision support systems and, increasingly, in clinical trial design strategies. The FDA has published an RWE framework that is quite detailed and likely very useful for study design and evidence generation.[25] From the standpoint of digital health ambition and hype, the ultimate goal of these types is to be able to use data as the sole basis of regulatory filings a practice often referred to as the use of synthetic patients.

Although still forward leaning, the concept of synthetic patients is becoming reality in clinical trials. The first successful use cases have been the use of synthetic control groups. Instead of collecting data from patients recruited for a trial who have been assigned to the control or standard-of-care arm, synthetic control arms model those comparators using real-world data that has previously been collected from sources such as health data generated during routine care, including electronic health records; administrative claims data; patient-generated data from fitness trackers or home medical equipment; disease registries; and historical clinical trial data.[26] The concept has been proven as Roche, for example, met European Union coverage requirements for marketing Alecensa (alectinib) in 20 European markets using a synthetic control arm. For patients, the benefit is the potential elimination of the risk of being assigned placebo instead of the test drug. This fear of placebo is a significant reason why some patients choose not to participate in trials. For the trial sponsor the benefits include reducing or eliminating the need to enroll control participants; a synthetic control arm can increase efficiency, reduce delays, lower trial costs, and speed lifesaving therapies to market.

Although the promise of new technologies is clear, it is hoped that this chapter has informed the reader about the exquisite level of specificity required in the design of each clinical trial, at each stage of development, for each type of medical product. These intricacies are often what is missed by big tech and small data and digital innovator companies alike. The assumption that overly simplistic approaches can "transform" clinical trials and medical product development is countered by high failure rates where 90% fail within two to five years.[27] The good news is that these high failure rates do not appear to be discouraging effort. Better news would be evidence that the newer efforts have actually learned from the failed or struggling efforts and do not simply repeat the same mistake of assuming that the Silicon Valley mantra of "move fast and break things" can be applied without modification to health care. The current, 2019, perspective of regulators was summed up very well by an FDA official during a Friends of Cancer Research meeting, "Using externally controlled data in places where today we are accepting single-arm studies is certainly better than single-arm studies," said Rajeshwari Sridhara, director of the FDA's Division of Biometrics V. "But we should not . . . say this is going to be the new standard and don't think about randomized, controlled studies."[28]

References

1. Lipinski CA, F Lombardo, BW Dominy, and PJ Feeney. Experimental and Computational Approaches to Estimate Solubility and Permeability in Drug Discovery and Development Settings. *Advanced Drug Delivery Reviews* 2001. 46(1–3):3–26.
2. Guha R. On Exploring Structure-Activity Relationships. *Methods in Molecular Biology* 2013. 993:81–94. doi:10.1007/978-1-62703-342-8_6
3. Wikipedia. The Human Genome Project. Accessed July 2019. https://en.wikipedia.org/wiki/Human_Genome_Project
4. Szymański P, M Markowicz, and E Mikiciuk-Olasik. Adaptation of High-Throughput Screening in Drug Discovery-Toxicological Screening Tests. *International Journal of Molecular Sciences* 2012. 13(1):427–452.
5. Wikipedia. Dirty Data. Accessed July 2019. https://en.wikipedia.org/wiki/Dirty_data
6. Mueller K. How to Clean Up Dirty Data in Patient Reported Outcomes. *SAS Conference Proceedings Online*. *PhUSE* 2010. https://www.lexjansen.com/phuse/2010/dh/DH02.pdf
7. U.S. Department of Health and Human Services FDA Center for Drug Evaluation and Research; U.S. Department of Health and Human Services FDA Center for Biologics Evaluation and Research; U.S. Department of Health and Human Services FDA Center

for Devices and Radiological Health. Guidance for Industry: Patient-Reported Outcome Measures: Use in Medical Product Development to Support Labeling Claims: Draft Guidance. *Health and Quality of Life Outcomes* 2006. 4:79. doi:10.1186/1477-7525-4-79

8. U.S. National Library of Medicine. ClinicalTrials.gov Background. https://clinicaltrials.gov/ct2/about-site/background

9. Hallinan ZP, KA Getz, and BE Bierer. Compliance with Results Reporting at ClinicalTrials.gov. *New England Journal of Medicine* 2015. 372(24):2370. doi:10.1056/NEJMc1504513

10. Kennet RS. Basic Concepts in the Statistical Design of Clinical Trials. Proceedings of a Workshop. 2003. Accessed July 2019. http://web.cs.elte.hu/probability/common/KPAClinTrials.PDF

11. Pannucci CJ, and EG Wilkins. Identifying and Avoiding Bias in Research. *Plastic and Reconstructive Surgery* 2010. 126(2):619–625. doi:10.1097/PRS.0b013e3181de24bc

12. Gluud LL. Bias in Clinical Intervention Research. *American Journal of Epidemiology* 2006. 163(6):493–501.

13. Krishnankutty B, S Bellary, NB Kumar, and LS Moodahadu. Data Management in Clinical Research: An Overview. *Indian Journal of Pharmacology* 2012. 44(2):168–172. doi:10.4103/0253-7613.93842

14. ClearData.com. Understanding GXP Regulations for Healthcare. Accessed September 2019. https://www.cleardata.com/wp-content/uploads/2018/01/GxP_Brochure_FINAL.pdf

15. Sylos M. The Top 5 Advantages of Software as a Service (SaaS). *IBM Blogs* 2013, September 18. Accessed August 2019. https://www.ibm.com/blogs/cloud-computing/2013/09/18/top-five-advantages-of-software-as-a-service-saas/

16. U.S. FDA. New Drug Application (NDA) 2019, June 10. Accessed August 2019. https://www.fda.gov/drugs/types-applications/new-drug-application-nda

17. ICH Guidance E6: Good Clinical Practice: Consolidated Guideline. US HHS, US FDA, CDER, CBER. 1996. [Last accessed on 2013, June 11]. No authors listed. Available from: http://www.fda.gov/downloads/Drugs/Guidances/ucm073122.pdf

18. U.S. FDA. 21CFR201.56. 2019, April 1. Accessed July 2019. https://www.accessdata.fda.gov/scripts/cdrh/cfdocs/cfcfr/CFRSearch.cfm?fr=201.56

19. U.S. FDA. How to Determine If Your Product Is a Medical Device. 2019, December 16. Accessed December 2019. https://www.fda.gov/medical-devices/classify-your-medical-device/product-medical-device

20. Faris O. Clinical Trials for Medical Devices: FDA and the IDE Process. Accessed December 2019. https://www.fda.gov/media/87603/download

21. Lehmann J. Drug and Medical Device Clinical Trials 101. 2016, October 19. Accessed November 2019. https://www.imarcresearch.com/blog/medical-device-clinical-trials-101

22. Borno HT, L Zhang, A Siegel, E Chang, and CJ Ryan. At What Cost to Clinical Trial Enrollment? A Retrospective Study of Patient Travel Burden in Cancer Clinical Trials. *The Oncologist*. 2018, April 26.

23. Institute of Medicine (U.S.) Forum on Drug Discovery, Development, and Translation. *Transforming Clinical Research in the United States: Challenges and Opportunities: Workshop Summary*. Washington, DC: National Academies Press, 2010.

24. U.S. FDA. Real-World Evidence. 2019, May 9. Accessed November 2019. https://www.fda.gov/science-research/science-and-research-special-topics/real-world-evidence

25. U.S. FDA. Framework for FDA's Real-World Evidence Program. 2018, December. Downloaded November 2019.

26. Goldsack J. Synthetic Control Arms Can Save Time and Money in Clinical Trials. *STAT*. 2019, February 5. Accessed November 2019.

27. The Medical Futurist. 10 Reasons Why Digital Startups Go Bust. 2019, March 14. Accessed November 2019. https://medicalfuturist.com/10-reasons-why-digital-health-startups-go-bust/

28. Sutter S. Pink Sheet—External Control ARMS: Better than Single ARM Studies but No Replacement for Randomization. 2019, January 2. Accessed November 2019. https://www.focr.org/news/pink-sheet-external-control-arms-better-single-arm-studies-no-replacement-randomization

7

Electronic Health Records

Promises, Progress, and Problems

American Recovery and Reinvestment Act and the Health Information Technology for Economic and Clinical Health Act

The American Recovery and Reinvestment Act (ARRA) was passed into law in February 2009 and was intended to support jobs and economic stability through the Great Recession of the late 2000s.[1] Among the investments were $19 billion for health information technology, primarily the implementation of electronic health records (EHRs) via the Health Information Technology for Economic and Clinical Health (HITECH) Act. The program was led by the Centers for Medicare and Medicaid Services (CMS) and the Office of the National Coordinator for Health Information Technology (ONC HIT). According to the Centers for Disease Control and Prevention (CDC), HITECH proposed the meaningful use of interoperable electronic health records throughout the U.S. healthcare delivery system as a critical national goal.[2]

Six years later, the total HITECH investment had surpassed $35.0 million and there were clear indications that the effort was struggling. Most notably, the fragmentation of the effort across too many EHR vendors and platforms led to gaps in interoperability—the key essential requirement to make a decentralized health system function. The ability to share medical record data, lab results, and other patient information across institutional boundaries via a secure network was always a stated goal but never mandated or even highlighted as an essential priority. Instead, Stage 1 of the meaningful use program failed to include any meaningful health information exchange requirements and lacked a vision to achieve interoperability, but it did incentivize the widespread adoption of EHR systems that providers now say are difficult to use and lack the ability to exchange information without costly upgrades.[3] This particular problem remains critical and unsolved at the time of this writing. The federal government continues to work on establishing interoperability and has launched additional efforts, such as the "Strategy

Digital Health. Eric D. Perakslis and Martin Stanley, Oxford University Press (2021). © Oxford University Press.
DOI: 10.1093/oso/9780197503133.003.0007

on Reducing Regulatory and Administrative Burden Relating to the Use of Health IT and EHRs" program in 2019, but progress remains elusive as many institutions have turned inward and are focused more on internal systems and strategy than on interoperability with their peers.[4]

Indeed, as I recently sat at one prestigious academic medical center in Boston, while scheduling surgery for a nonhealing compound tibial-fibula fracture, I watched as the nurse practitioner tried in vain to pull up my records from my primary institution a few miles down the road using an interface allegedly designed exactly for this purpose. Similarly, I have completely failed at assembling my own records via the patient portals of these two institutions. One institution posts radiology reports in the "Your Results" section of their My Chart patient portal but the other does not. Assembling my data in one place required the creation of multiple accounts, e-mails, and faxes. Unfortunately, this is considered the norm for health data interoperability in October 2019, 10 years after the HITECH Act went into effect.

Meaningful Use was intended to ensure the use of certified EHR technology in a "meaningful" manner (e.g., electronic prescribing); ensuring that the certified EHR technology provides for the electronic exchange of health information to improve the quality of care. By using certified EHR technology, the provider must submit to the Secretary of Health & Human Services (HHS) information on the quality of care and other measures. The concept of meaningful use rested on the five pillars of health outcomes policy priorities, namely:

1. Improve quality, safety, and efficiency, as well as reduce health disparities
2. Engage patients and families in their health
3. Improve care coordination
4. Improve population and public health
5. Ensure adequate privacy and security protection for personal health information.

These goals were intended to be delivered via a three-stage approach:

- Stage 1 set the foundation by establishing requirements for the electronic capture of clinical data, including providing patients with electronic copies of health information.
- Stage 2 expanded upon the Stage 1 criteria with a focus on advancing clinical processes and ensuring that the meaningful use of EHRs supported the aims and priorities of the National Quality Strategy. Stage 2 criteria encouraged the use of Certified EHR Technology (CEHRT) for

continuous quality improvement at the point of care and the exchange of information in the most structured format possible.

- In October 2015, CMS released a final rule that established Stage 3 in 2017 and beyond, which focused on using CEHRT to improve health outcomes. In addition, this rule modified Stage 2 to ease reporting requirements and align with other CMS programs.

The way this was actually intended to work, and incentivize medical record adoption and use, was that technical capabilities were directly tied to payment incentives via a points system. For example, according to the Proposed Scoring Methodology for Quality Payment Program (QPP), having electronic subscribing capability (e-subscribing) is worth 5 points, support of electronic patient referral loops via the electronic transfer of data is worth 20 points, providing patients electronic access to their own medical data is worth 40 points, etc. These task-based automation incentives led to exactly what nobody wanted or expected, a reformatting of clinical encounters from patient-care-focused to data-entry-dominant. The current state is almost chaotic. At the time of this writing, the current estimates are that more than $39 billion has been invested to date on EHR implementation with little patient or provider benefit to show for it. Among the dozens of reported downsides, out of control costs, unknown patient safety risks, and clinician burnout top the lists.[5]

Outcomes, status, and unintended consequences

The majority of EHR complaints have their basis in the time-consuming and inflexible ways most EHR systems work. To understand them, it is important to understand their genesis was not based in medical practice or research, but in simplifying medical billing. In our U.S. fee-for-service medical system, one of the most effective ways to build a longitudinal record of a patient journey is to simply tally up the consults, diagnostics, and procedures that a patient receives each time they present in the care setting. Although this workflow is great at tallying fees, it does not mimic ideal clinical workflow nor does it capture the reasons or rationale behind any of the listed occurrences. The result of any rigid multiple-choice and form-based computer application is often that a lot of important data, as viewed by the entering clinician, is either force-fitted into the "best" multiple choice answer or listed as free text within the notes section of the EHR. Neither of these is ideal, especially from the standpoint of making the records understandable to the next clinician who accesses the patient chart.

Another unintended consequence of the ARRA EHR investments has been fiscal strain. Taken as a whole industry, the average annual support cost for software systems runs about 30% of the original purchase price. This means that a new software system that costs a million dollars to procure and implement will cost roughly $300,000 per year to keep running. There are variances, but under 15% is very rare and over 40% would be considered poor performance. With respect to EHRs, the upfront licensing costs alone (not including implementation, data migration, compliance, server hardware, etc.) have averaged from $1.200 to $500,000 with ongoing costs averaging $200 to more than $35,000; the hidden costs, however, can be much, much higher.[6] The original intent was that the implementations would be subsidized by ARRA and the ongoing costs would be fully covered via reimbursement incentives from CMS, but this has not been the case in many instances. Indeed, the only comprehensive review at the time of this writing was unable to confirm the predicted cost benefits of EHRs.[7] It is also important to note that costs and value varied widely as each medical system selected and implemented its own solution. The variance in performance appears significant with several notable, but high-profile outliers, such as the announcement by the MD Anderson Cancer Center that they needed to cut 900 jobs due to cost overruns from their EHR implementation.[8] Although outliers such as this grab attention, the more common truth is that, in my experience, many institutions struggle with the costs of EHR management. Cost concerns, combined with usability and productivity issues, result in systems that are unpopular at most institutions. The path forward is unclear. The cost of reverting back to paper would not be covered by an ARRA-type initiative, at least not today. Hence, many in clinical care feel trapped and held hostage by these systems.

With respect to patient safety, the scorecard is mixed. One study examined perceptions around the impacts of EHRs on patient safety and yielded mixed results, some of which pointed to issues that may be caused more by EHR implementation than by the EHR system itself.[9] These elements are important, given that there is growing evidence that the types of workarounds that can occur as a result of EHR implementations can actually increase patient safety risks.[10, 11] For example, the use of "copy and paste" functions within these systems has been linked with increased patient safety risks.[12] Indeed, this particular finding is important for many elements of digital health, because data management is an unavoidable adjuvant. There is a great deal of work still to be done.

The rise of an industrial-medical complex

One of the most profound conversations I had in my first few weeks at the FDA was with a senior fellow. These types of folks are often the wisest and most insightful you can meet in any organization. Typically, they are very experienced, know the institutions extremely well, and exist primarily as individual contributor mentors to those in leadership. My challenge, in his words, would be to fend off the vendor industrial complex that he claimed really "ran IT for the federal government." He wasn't wrong. Vivek Kundra, who served as the first Chief Information Officer (CIO) of the United States from March 2009 until August 2011 under President Barack Obama, made similar observations in his excellent *25 Point Plan to Reform Federal Information Technology Management*.[13] In his plan, Vivek called for multiple actions to improve procurement and vendor management. He understood that these relationships determined almost all elements of technology service, and that accountability had to be established.

Wikipedia defines an industrial complex as a socioeconomic concept wherein businesses become entwined in social or political systems or institutions, creating or bolstering a profit economy from these systems. Such a complex is said to pursue its own financial interests regardless of, and often at the expense of, the best interests of society and individuals. Businesses within an industrial complex may have been created to advance a social or political goal, but they mostly profit when the goal is not reached. The industrial complex may profit financially from maintaining socially detrimental or inefficient systems.[14] Many, the authors included, feel that this definition applies well to the EHR marketplace.

As early as 2012, it was very clear that Epic, a Wisconsin-based EHR company was on its way to a majority of market share. Epic, founded in a basement in 1979 with one and a half employees, develops software to help people get well, help people stay well, and help future generations be healthier—all according to their website.[15] At that time, David Shaywitz foresaw the possibility and wrote in *The Atlantic*, "most of the nation's largest and most prestigious medical centers seem headed towards a relatively closed health information system, driven by a single dominant private company, Wisconsin-based Epic, which excels at the near-flawless, customized installation of their client-server platform in big hospitals."[16] He was right. Seven years later, healthcare technology interoperability is still no more than a distant goal and the number of EHR vendors has dropped from more than 1,000 to less than 400.[17] This has left clinicians concerned about the financial implications of fee increases, increased support costs, or the expense of having to migrate to a new system if their current vendor is acquired or closes down. From the practice perspective, many of the remaining EHRs exist because they supply niche, often specialty-specific, capabilities.

Despite clinician concerns and calls for greatly improved interoperability and affordability, it does appear that a true medical industrial complex has arisen in the EHR marketplace and that change, improvement, or reform are not in sight. Currently just two companies, EPIC and Cerner, hold 85% of the large hospital market, with EPIC alone holding 58%. More than 90 merger and acquisition (M&A) deals occurred in the EHR marketplace in 2018 alone.[18]

It is important to note that the large players are not at all solely responsible for the interoperability issues, although they clearly need to be part of the fix. For example, hospitals are large, complex, and matrixed organizations with networks of affiliates beyond their walls. Despite market consolidation by core EHR products, many hospitals still have an average of 10 different EHRs in use across their affiliate and outpatient organizations. It is considered unlikely that the most specialized of these systems will ever be consolidated into a single core product. Hence, the complex is highly dichotomous, complex, interdependent, and very difficult to influence.

Beyond the varied marketplace, it is also important to understand that each EHR implementation is far more custom than might be expected. Different historical systems and preexisting technology stacks, as well as numbers and types of specialty practices and care are just a few of the dozens of reasons that one implementation of a system such as EPIC may struggle to connect with another. To its credit, EPIC is taking steps to make individual implementations of its system compatible with one another via a "One Virtual System Worldwide" initiative aimed at combining functionalities and data from across varying EPIC ecosystems. "We're taking interoperability from being able to 'view more' to being able to 'do more,'" said Dave Fuhrmann, EPIC Vice President of Interoperability in a statement. "Over the last decade we expanded the amount of data that customers can exchange, going well beyond industry requirements. Now, our new functionality 'Working Together' will allow clinicians to work across EPIC organizations to improve the care for their patients."[19]

Lastly, a massive after-market for healthcare data is growing exponentially within the health IT industrial complex and, with mixed results, it is simultaneously trying to optimize the utility and value of healthcare data. Attempts to map this marketplace yield a ridiculously complex picture.[20]

With respect to the larger ecosystem, EHRs are only one point of origination for healthcare data. There are many others including pharmacies, laboratories, medical imaging facilities, payers, government agencies, and socioeconomic data sources. Much of this data is actively being monetized to support research and commercialization of medical process via mechanisms that include data aggregators and brokers, analytics and knowledge management companies, and academic labs, as well as private and public partnerships and consortia. On the surface, these are well-intentioned enterprises looking to improve patient care and the overall efficacy of the healthcare system. Deeper study, however, reveals a complex web of questionable business models and incentives, especially from the standpoint of patient data rights, healthcare fragmentation, and challenges to technology standardization. Indeed, many of the companies and consortia described later started off trying to reduce healthcare fragmentation only to quickly become the latest silo to end all silos. Beyond market dynamics, the greater concerns are patient rights and privacy.

Patients as data owners

As previously discussed, the concepts of data ownership in health care are quite complex. First, actual "ownership" of health care data is regulated at the state level in the United States. Generally, when health information is captured and documented in written or electronic form, and because the health care provider owns the media in which the information is recorded and stored, the health care provider gains property rights over possession of data.[21] Patients have privacy, accuracy, and security rights under HIPAA and state law but not, really, ownership. This is not as bad as it may seem at first glance, because the concepts of ownership within our society are complex.

Ownership infers rights but also obligations and liabilities. According to the Brookings Institute,

> Treating data like it is property fails to recognize either the value that varieties of personal information serve or the abiding interest that individuals have in their personal information even if they choose to "sell" it. Data is not a commodity. It is information. Any system of information rights—whether patents, copyrights, and other intellectual property, or privacy rights—presents some tension with strong interest in the free flow of information that is reflected by the First Amendment. Our personal information is in demand precisely because it has value to others and

to society across a myriad of uses. Treating personal information as property to be licensed or sold may induce people to trade away their privacy rights for very little value while injecting enormous friction into free flow of information. The better way to strengthen privacy is to ensure that individual privacy interests are respected as personal information flows to desirable uses, not to reduce personal data to a commodity."[22]

But how to do this in practice? The truth is that health data is being traded and treated as a commodity, but individual patient records are not a commodity. One enabler, or culprit depending on your point of view, are the strategies around anonymization and/or deidentification. If patients do not own their data but are entitled to have their privacy and security protected, does separating the data from the identity of each/any patient ensure those protections? The health data complex thinks so. In fact, many of the players in healthcare data use this deidentification as a model to enable a secondary business selling the data from their primary business. For example, a contract laboratory that deidentifies lab results and sells population-level, or even patient-level, data. On the surface, this appears harmless, but this is far from the case. First, none of the techniques used to deidentify health data is perfect and most are easily foiled by modern computing power and algorithms.[23,24] Next, according to Boris Lubarsky at Georgetown Law, 'There is no comprehensive data privacy law in America—it is regulated on an ad-hoc industry-by-industry basis. None of this patchwork of laws and regulations sets limits on the use or sale of "anonymized" data. There is no duty to report if data has been re-identified. There is no private cause of action for an individual seeking redress for re-identified data, and no external way to verify if a private entity has privately de-identified "anonymized" data exists. The theory that data scrubbed of personally identifying information cannot be re-identified has time and again been shown to no longer hold true. Our current ad-hoc approach is antiquated and inadequate for addressing the new technological challenges re-identified data presents.[25]

This is extremely important in healthcare, given that medical data contains vulnerabilities that could be used in a prejudicial way against patients.

These types of concerns were the drivers of the Genetic Nondiscrimination Act. The Genetic Information Nondiscrimination Act (GINA) of 2008 protects Americans from discrimination based on their genetic information in both health insurance (Title I) and employment (Title II). Title I amends the Employee Retirement Income Security Act of 1974 (ERISA), the Public Health Service Act (PHSA), and the Internal Revenue Code (IRC), through the Health Insurance Portability and Accountability Act of 1996 (HIPAA), as well as the Social Security Act, to prohibit health insurers from engaging in genetic discrimination.[26] GINA represents the successful case of creating legislation in a timely manner with respect to technology development. During the human genome project, experts foresaw the vulnerabilities that genetic data could cause and took action. This has not happened with respect to healthcare data, but it is desperately needed because many feel that patient-centered data control is the key to better health data interoperability and, more importantly, to better care.

As described by Mandl and Kohane in the *New England Journal of Medicine* in 2016,

A patient-controlled health-record infrastructure can support the development of highly desirable health system qualities. First, it allows a patient to effectively become a health information exchange of one: as data accumulate in a patient-controlled repository, a complete picture of the patient emerges. If patients can obtain their data wherever they go, they can share them with physicians as needed—rather than vice versa. We believe the Meaningful Use program would have been more successful if it had rewarded clinicians for storing data in patient-controlled repositories rather than in EHRs that fragment data across the health care system.[27]

This call has indeed been heard and, in some ways, answered by federal regulators who increasingly see patient "ownership" of health data as the solution to THE interoperability problem, although much of their effort has focused on programming interfaces (APIs) and standards.[28] Although these approaches would likely ease the technical challenges of data interoperability, they do not at all address the social challenges previously discussed. Indeed, the API approach is likely to exacerbate the privacy and autonomy challenges. According to Mandl, Gottleib, and Mandel, HIPAA does not adequately address the issue. It does allow an app developer to become a business associate of a covered entity (such as a provider or healthcare institution), but this arrangement only applies when an app is managing health information on behalf of the covered entity—whereas in a consumer-centric ecosystem, many apps will choose to have a relationship with a consumer directly. Importantly, the covered entity itself may be a conflicted party when the patient wishes to use an app that either (1) shares data with a competing healthcare provider or (2) competes with the functionality of the entity's EHR. These conflicts could limit data flow across institutions and raise the barrier to entry for new, innovative applications. Further, the HIPAA business associate framework *does not* prevent commercial use of patient's data without consent. Indeed, there is still a great deal of work to be done.

References

1. Congress.gov. H.R.1 – American Recovery and Reinvestment Act of 2009. 2009. Accessed July 2019. https://www.congress.gov/bill/111th-congress/house-bill/1
2. CDC. Public Health and Promoting Interoperability Programs (formerly, known as Electronic Health Records Meaningful Use). 2019, September 9. Accessed October 2019. https://www.cdc.gov/ehrmeaningfuluse/introduction.html
3. Thune J et al. Where is HITECH's 35 Billion Dollar Investment Going? *Health Affairs Blog.* 2015, March 4. https://www.healthaffairs.org/do/10.1377/hblog20150304.045199/full/
4. Office of the National Coordinator for Health Information Technology. Strategy on Reducing Regulatory and Administrative Burden Relating to the Use of Health IT and EHRs. Draft for Public Comment. November 2018.
5. Schulte F, and E Fry. Death By 1,000 Clicks: Where Electronic Health Records Went Wrong. *Kaiser Health News.* 2019, March 18.
6. Dyrda L. 18 Hidden Costs in EHR Purchase and Implementation. *Becker's Health IT and CIO Report.* 2016, December 16.
7. Reis ZSN, TA Maia, MS Marcolino, F Becerra-Posada, D Novillo-Ortiz, and ALP Ribeiro. Is The Evidence of Cost Benefits of Electronic Medical Records, Standards, or Interoperability in Hospital Information Systems? Overview of Systematic Reviews. *JMIR Medical Informatics* 2017. 5(3):e26.
8. Castellucci M. MD Anderson Cancer Center to Cut 900 Jobs Due to Losses from EHR Rollout. *Modern Healthcare.* 2017, January 6.
9. Wang MD, R Khanna, and N Najafi. Characterizing the Source of Text in Electronic Health Record Progress Notes. *JAMA Internal Medicine* 2017. 177(8):1212–1213.
10. Tubaishat A. The Effect of Electronic Health Records on Patient Safety: A Qualitative Exploratory Study. *Informatics for Health and Social Care* 2019. 44(1):79–91.
11. Garbhart T. The Impact of Electronic Health Records in Patient Safety. *Compass Clinical Consulting* 2019, January 4. Accessed October 2019. https://www.compass-clinical.com/electronic-health-record-patient-safety/
12. Kent J. Pew: EHR Usability Concerns May Still Impact Patient Safety. HealthITAnalytics. 2017, December 21. Accessed November 2019. https://healthitanalytics.com/news/pew-ehr-usability-concerns-may-still-impact-patient-safety
13. Kundra V. 25 Point Implementation Plan to Reform Federal Information Technology Management. 2010, December 9. https://www.dhs.gov/sites/default/files/publications/digital-strategy/25-point-implementation-plan-to-reform-federal-it.pdf
14. Wikipedia. Industrial Complex. Accessed July 2019. https://en.wikipedia.org/wiki/Industrial_complex
15. EPIC.com. About EPIC. Accessed July 2019. https://www.epic.com/about
16. Shaywitz D. Is One Company About to Lock Up the Electronic Medical Records Market? *The Atlantic.* 2012, June 14.
17. Pratt MK. EHR Market Consolidation and the Impact on Physicians. *Medical Economics.* 2019, January 2.
18. LaRock Z. How Epic and Cerner Will Retain Control of the EHR Market. *Business Insider.* 2019, May 6.
19. Pennic J. EPIC Launches One Virtual System Worldwide to Support Interoperability. 2018, January 31. Accessed November 2019. https://hitconsultant.net/2018/01/31/epic-launches-one-virtual-system-worldwide-interoperability/#.XadJgZNKjOQ
20. Datavant. The Fragmentation of Health Data. 2019, September. Accessed November 2019. https://datavant.com/2018/08/01/the-fragmentation-of-health-data/
21. Sharma R. Who Really Owns Your Health Data? *Forbes.* 2018, April 23.

22. Kerry CF, and JB Morris. Why Data Ownership Is the Wrong Approach to Protecting Privacy. Brookings Institute. 2019, June 26. Accessed November 2019. https://www.brookings.edu/blog/techtank/2019/06/26/why-data-ownership-is-the-wrong-approach-to-protecting-privacy/

23. Cohen JK. AI Can Re-Identify De-Identified Health Data, Study Finds. *Becker's Hospital Review*. 2019, January 3.

24. Dark Daily. Researchers Easily Reidentify Deidentified Patient Records with 95% Accuracy; Privacy Protection of Patient Test Records a Concern for Clinical Laboratories. 2018, October 10. Accessed August 2019. https://www.darkdaily.com/researchers-easily-reidentify-deidentified-patient-records-with-95-accuracy-privacy-protection-of-patient-test-records-a-concern-for-clinical-laboratories/

25. Lubarsky B. Re-Identification of "Anonymized Data". *Georgetown Law Review*. 2017, 1 GEO. L. TECH. REV. 202 April.

26. NIH Genome.gov. National Human Genome Research Institute. *Genetic Discrimination*. 2020, January 16. Accessed January 2020. https://www.genome.gov/about-genomics/policy-issues/Genetic-Discrimination

27. Mandl KD, and IS Kohane. Time for a Patient-Driven Health Information Economy? *New England Journal of Medicine* 2016. 374(3):205–208.

28. Ellis A. New Report Available: Push Button Health: Advancing SMART/HL7 Bulk Data Export/FLAT FHIR. SMARThealthIT.org. 2019, December 16. Accessed December 2019. https://smarthealthit.org/an-app-platform-for-healthcare/news/

PART 2

THE 10 TOXICITIES
OF DIGITAL HEALTH

8

Introducing the 10 Toxicities

Understanding the 10 Toxicities of Digital Health

Direct-to-consumer (DTC) drug marketing advertisements are tightly regulated and even the most tasteless DTC ads must clearly disclose all known potential side effects. The same is not yet true for digital health technologies, but this needs to change. In an age of rampant medical misinformation and declining public trust in medicine and science, the touting of expensive and unproven medical technologies is a risk to public health. The issue is exacerbated by what can only be described as some form of blind spot with respect to this topic. As a devout follower of medical science on Twitter, I am struck when I see clinicians of true social media influencer status tweet excitedly, "Alexa, now HIPAA-compliant" (which does nothing to ensure privacy) without any caution of potential hazards of use or implications for personal privacy. I never see these same clinicians touting a newly approved drug or newly released clinical study without a balanced view of limitations or potential adverse events (AEs).

As someone who has been delivering new technologies into clinical care since 1985, I feel this is at least partially my fault. Until we study, validate, and list the potential side effects of digital health tools, the potential hazards cannot be understood or communicated. This issue is especially important because many new medical technologies, be they digital tools or at-home screening tests for certain cancer, are being marketed directly to consumers. As we discussed earlier, the first legal use of caveat emptor, the principle that the buyer alone is responsible for determining the suitability and quality of goods prior to purchase, was a case of medical "technology." In 1603 in *Chandelor v Lupus*, a man accused a seller of selling him a false bezoar stone, a stone that forms in the intestines of animals and is alleged to have magical healing properties. The stone turned out to not be a bezoar stone, but the court ruled that the buyer had no right to a refund unless he could prove deceit or violation of a warranty, which the buyer could not do.[1] The chapters that follow within this section list potential digital bezoar stones, and we should

Digital Health. Eric D. Perakslis and Martin Stanley, Oxford University Press (2021). © Oxford University Press.
DOI: 10.1093/oso/9780197503133.003.0008

begin to think carefully about how we message advancements in digital health within the context of very real risks.

In thinking through the risks, threats, and resulting toxicities, an obvious opportunity for classification is whether or not the risks and threats are derived from human malfeasance. According to NIST, an adversary is an individual, group, organization, or government that conducts or has the intent to conduct detrimental activities.[2] A detailed understanding of the specific type of adversary for each type of risk further illuminates the potential impact if the adversary is successful in its nefarious ends. For example, the motivations of one adversary may amount to simple theft, but the motivation of another might be reputational harm against a healthcare institution. Both are clear, present, and common risks, but one is a risk to patient confidentiality and the other is a risk to availability of care, and as such, the mitigations are necessarily unique. Because the nature of adversarial activity is fundamental to the nature of the resulting risks and mitigations, we have categorized each specific toxicity as adversarially driven or not.

Lastly, it is important to admit up front that this categorization is imperfect. It has the potential to change over time along with the healthcare environment, and because it is contextual, it will apply most but not all of the time. In fact, the most common cases where the categorizations are imperfect may be the most important of all, due to the complexities that arise when both adversarial and nonadversarial components exist. For example, as we will discuss, social media use has been blamed for contributing to mental stresses such as loneliness, envy, and depression. For the most part, these appear to be nonadversarial in nature. These platforms, however, are also among the most prolific sources of medical misinformation, which is often adversarially driven. As a result, social media risks should be studied in each context individually and also as an aggregate summation.

References

1. Wikipedia. *Chandelor v Lupus*. Accessed July 2019. https://en.wikipedia.org/wiki/Chandelor_v_Lopus
2. NIST. Computer Security Resource Center. Accessed July 2020. https://csrc.nist.gov/glossary/term/adversary

9

Adversarially Driven Toxicities

Cybercrime

As a society, we have seen the devastating and debilitating impact that cyberattacks, such as WannaCry, can have on healthcare systems. It should be well-recognized that healthcare cybersecurity is an essential element of patient safety. Despite the fact that the use of digital healthcare devices and Internet-connected technologies exposes the human body to these risks, healthcare-specific precautions are not yet mandated by anyone. This must change, and these types of potential harms must be factored explicitly within medical benefit-risk determinations. Types of cyberattacks and cybercrime focused on health care specifically include hacks that disrupt clinical care, as well as theft of personal financial information, theft of personal health information, theft of medical research, and terrorism. Although the nature and likelihood of these threats is becoming better understood, the potential impacts to individual patients is not.

In regard to physical harm, Internet and patient-connected medical devices can be hacked, which can lead to disruption of use, false readings, and malfunction.[1] Other forms of cybercrime based on stolen or falsified patient and provider data include identity theft and insurance fraud; medical licensing fraud to forge prescriptions; insurance fraud; drug counterfeiting and/or smuggling; and nefarious use of biometric data.[2] These crimes are clearly worrisome, but in the author's experience, most patients, providers, and health technology companies are unaware of how common they are. In 2016, *Consumer Reports* detailed these types of crimes and the difficulties the victims encountered restoring their reputations.[3] In one case, two years after the incident, a victim of identity theft received a call from a bail bondsman just before she was about to be arrested for acquiring more than 1,700 opioid-painkiller pills through local pharmacies. According to the victim, "I had my mug shot taken, my fingerprints taken." The victim suffered from psoriasis, and she was so stressed that she broke out in the signature rash. "The policemen looked at my hands and said: That's what drug users' hands look like." They just assumed I was guilty." These types of stories have become

Digital Health. Eric D. Perakslis and Martin Stanley, Oxford University Press (2021). © Oxford University Press.
DOI: 10.1093/oso/9780197503133.003.0009

commonplace and anyone who has tried to clear even a single incorrect entry on their credit report understands how financially debilitating cybercrime can be. Apologies for the terrible pun, but health care must literally stop the bleeding when it comes to cybercrime.

Privacy

Personal privacy faces significant challenges in the surveillance economy, and there is a massive amount of work to be done with respect to personal privacy and digital health. In short, the principle of caveat emptor must be diligently applied here. The default setting of the Internet is "open." It is that simple. End user license agreements and "terms of use" are typically not privacy assurance vehicles, and, unless there are additional explicit assurances of privacy, consumers must assume that their data is being captured and shared with third parties, including employers, insurers, and law enforcement agencies.

Although it is easy to assume that privacy is important and more privacy is better than less privacy, meaningful change will only happen if the reasons why privacy are important become the focus. According to Daniel Solove, the founder of TeachPrivacy, privacy is essential in maintaining: a limit on the power of government and private sector companies; respect for individuals and individual preferences; a tool for reputation management for institutions and individuals; appropriate social, ethical, and legal boundaries; trust; control and self-determination; freedom of thought and speech; freedom of and for social and political activities; the ability for individuals and institutions to change and have second chances; the ability of not having to explain oneself and to not be judged from afar by those with incomplete knowledge.[4]

Looking at Solove's list, one observes that privacy is really not about one thing but many. Privacy has been compared to the environment: "It's about too many things to be useful, so everybody ends up trampling it for a host of petty reasons. Leading to a world that's degraded and hostile, and that would never have been chosen had the consequences been made clear."[5] Not a bad metaphor given that privacy is clearly a set of motivations and concerns versus a single tangible idea. If we were to sift out one single essence of the importance of privacy in our lives, it probably should be control. The fact is that we don't really know who is seeing our data or how they're using it. Even the people whose business it is to know don't know.[6] If for no other reason, privacy must be assured so that individuals know how their interests are being managed and how their information is being used, especially in health care. Further, the consequence of lost privacy is that it stays lost, forever.

One of the reasons that privacy is such an issue in health care is because of the long-standing "nothing to hide" arguments being made, primarily by the human surveillance industrial complex. The idea here is that privacy is overvalued and that many public goods come from an open and underregulated data economy. I frequently have heard the proposition that health care could be revolutionized and clinical trials made unnecessary if all health data were shared. Frankly, it is simply naivete' from well-meaning (and I do believe that) individuals who do not understand sociology, the scientific method, or basic biostatistics. Indeed, Glenn Greenwald, one of the first reporters to see—and write about—the Edward Snowden files, offers a great example and quote: "Over the last 16 months, as I've debated this issue around the world, every single time somebody has said to me, 'I don't really worry about invasions of privacy because I don't have anything to hide.' I always say the same thing to them. I get out a pen, I write down my email address. I say, "Here's my email address. What I want you to do when you get home is email me the passwords to all of your email accounts, not just the nice, respectable work one in your name, but all of them, because I want to be able to just troll through what it is you're doing online, read what I want to read and publish whatever I find interesting. After all, if you're not a bad person, if you're doing nothing wrong, you should have nothing to hide.' Not a single person has taken me up on that offer."[7,8]

Looking into the potential and common harms from privacy loss, specifically healthcare privacy breaches, most common impacts include identity theft and fraud.[9] One study in the *Annals of Internal Medicine* studied more than 1,500 HHS cyber breach claims that occurred over 10 years. Patient data was categorized by demographic details, service or financial data, and medical information. Within these categories, the researchers focused on the data most likely to be exploited for fraud. HIV status, substance abuse, cancer, and other sensitive diagnoses were classified as the most sensitive information based on privacy implications. The researchers found that 194 breaches, or 66%, exposed sensitive demographic information such as Social Security numbers, dates of birth, or driver's license numbers, impacting 150 million patients. Meanwhile, 71% of breaches affecting 159 million patients exposed demographic or financial information, which put those patients at risk of fraud or identity theft. The data included billing amounts, payment data, service dates, and other related metrics. Just 2% of the breaches analyzed by researchers exposed medical information, such as diagnoses. This small percentage, however, impacted 2.4 million patients. Furthermore, 65% compromised general clinical or medical information, which impacted 48 million patients. These numbers are staggering and demonstrate the high value of healthcare data as a target along with the likelihood that medicine is a high-probability vector for identity theft.

Precise quantification of the problem is difficult, because disclosures often are kept as private as possible, and because many institutions may not recognize breaches for months or years after they happen. Specifically, the Ponemon 2017 Cost of Data Breach Study determined that U.S. companies took an average of 206 days to detect a data breach and that this time frame was getting longer, not shorter, year on year.[10] By all accounts, the problem is severe, extensive, and not getting better. Further, in addition to the high volume and high probability of personal data being compromised within the healthcare system, there are a number of reasons why healthcare data breaches have greater consequences than financial data breaches. Specifically, victims of healthcare data breaches have fewer resources to help them. For instance, free identity monitoring offered when health records are breached remedies financial impacts of the breach rather than the compromise of medical records.[11] Other healthcare data breach specific consequences include lack of adequate recompense to victims, ever-increasing risks due to lack of controls over the propagation of medical technologies, and the potentially deadly consequences of perpetrators who manipulate and change victims' data to seek medical services for themselves. This may sound far-fetched, but the 2013 Ponemon Survey on Medical Identity Theft found that most victims are unaware that medical identity theft can create inaccuracies in their permanent medical records and that these inaccuracies can have severe or deadly consequences.[12] (A change in a patient's blood type offers a good example of such an inaccuracy.) The benefits of privacy and cybersecurity of health information are quite different than the commonly understood benefits associated with protecting financial data. The consequences of breached health information can be dire, and the preventative controls and necessary urgency are simply not being applied by most institutions. To be frank, these risks really should be disclosed in the same ways that other healthcare risks are discussed with patients.

Will privacy law in the United States improve? At the time of this writing, a great number of calls have gone out for stronger privacy regulations to protect consumers and patients. With GDPR in effect for more than 18 months and the California Consumer Privacy Act (CCPA) having gone into effect on January 1, 2020, there are plenty of exemplars of solid and far more modern privacy regulations than those currently in effect in the United States.[13] Several options are currently on the table. The Consumer Online Privacy Act, introduced by Democratic Senator Maria Cantwell, proposes:

- Consumers would have the right to view, correct, and delete their data. They theoretically would also be able to stop it from being sold third parties.
- Companies could face higher fines for data abuse.
- Companies could be fined for first-time privacy offenses.
- Companies would be forced to obtain special permission to collect sensitive data. This would include location information, biometrics, and other information that can't be easily changed, such as a password.
- The Federal Trade Commission could expand with the creation of a bureau for privacy.
- A data security fund would be established, to be run by the Treasury Department.
- State attorneys general would be allowed to bring privacy lawsuits under federal law.
- Companies would be required to audit their algorithms for bias—especially with regard to financial discrimination or housing.[14]

In this proposed legislation, the provision for special permission to collect sensitive data such as location and biometrics would be extremely important for the issues of patient privacy and security, because, by definition, digital health sensors are biometric measurement, storage, and transmission devices.

Concurrently, at the time of this writing, there is also a Senate bill being introduced by Republican Roger Wicker. According to Reuters, this bill would set nationwide rules for handling of personal information online and elsewhere and override state laws, including California's law set to take effect next year.[15] This issue, that of state-based privacy laws, is representative of the complexity associated with regulating privacy at the national level. It is easy to understand and empathize with states' rights to protect their citizens as they best feel fit, but there are also clear national consequences that must be considered. For example, according to Michael Beckerman in his *New York Times* opinion piece on the subject,

> The risk is that Americans have a false sense of security that their privacy is consistently protected. The cost is that online and offline businesses large and small pay a steep price to comply with a vast array of privacy rules. A patchwork of state laws means that a California woman who orders an item from a Missouri business that manufactures in Florida could have her data regulated by three separate laws, or by no applicable law. Despite California's Consumer Privacy Protection Act the state's residents cannot be assured that the protections that apply when they deal with a business covered by the law will apply when they shop at their corner store, travel

across the country or engage in online transactions with companies that are not subject to California's privacy law.[16]

At the time of this writing, 26 states are considering, debating, or have already passed state-based privacy regulation.[17] Mr. Beckerman clearly has a point, although there is a great deal to consider on both sides of this issue. The authors feel the current state of affairs, despite being in such dramatic flux, represents an unacceptable risk of harm to patients and the medical system as a whole. We will continue the dialogue by discussing what we feel good privacy law should accomplish.

What does good health data privacy look like in the age of digital health? As previously discussed, healthcare and consumer data privacy are hot topics with new ideas, opinions, and risks appearing weekly if not daily. Out of the noise, a few strong opinions and ideas stand out. Most notably, an excellent *Health Affairs* (HA) piece by Lisa Bari and Daniel P. O'Neil, which we will explore in detail.[18] Bari and O'Neil propose five steps to modernize HIPPA:

1. "Define individually identifiable health information as an inherently protected class of data, rather than a class that is protected only when created or held by certain entities." This would help close a significant number of loopholes currently being exploited by health data market brokers and similar, as it simply does not make sense that healthcare providers are held to a higher standard than nonhealthcare providers when it comes to the exact same data on the exact same people.
2. "Create new definitions of individually identifiable health information 'custodians' and 'processors,' whose obligations (and liability) are like those of covered entities and business associates under existing law."
3. "Establish individuals' right to access, amend, and delete individually identifiable health information that is held by a custodian or processor, and to know about and control the use or disclosure of their own data, including any participation in de-identified data sets used for research purposes." This is also very important. Much of the secondary health data market assumes there is no chance of harm, so no liability at all, if data has been anonymized. Given the ease with which virtually all deidentification approaches have been compromised, along with the fact that deidentified data can be quickly reidentified when mixed with additional data, there are really no patient protections in these approaches. Nor is there recourse if harm happens. This proposal indeed closes an important gap.

4. "Codify the **permitted uses** of such individually identifiable health information, absent explicit, ongoing, and granular patient consent. These use categories could be rooted in the fiduciary principle that already applies to clinicians and other professionals with a duty of care and might correspond to the 'treatment' use cases in existing regulations. A heart rate monitor worn for fitness could, for example, be permitted to use the data to share personalized, clinically validated health information for the patient's benefit, but could not use the same data to power targeted advertising, which would benefit the company that produces the monitor."

5. "Specify clear parameters for consumer-friendly and revocable consent, for any use or disclosure of data beyond the narrowly permitted categories above." Although this is an enviable goal, many healthcare providers feel that the ethical informed consent principles and practices that serve so well in human subjects research are simply not applicable to the care-delivery environment. Indeed, it is tricky. We will have to see if this comes together and can be accomplished reasonably.

With respect to implementation path, Bari and O'Neil suggest:

"To extend the existing HIPAA security and breach notification rules to the new custodians and processors, legislators should focus on three steps:

1. Apply the existing security rule to all custodians and processors of individually identifiable health information, irrespective of the data provenance or primary customer.

2. Require all custodians and processors to directly notify individuals, the media, and the HHS secretary in the event of a breach. Processors that are acting as business associates of a covered entity would also remain obligated to notify that covered entity of the breach.

3. Establish specific, consumer-friendly, and granular notification requirements. These notifications would specify which data elements were inappropriately exposed to whom and would be designed for easy public comprehension and directly linked to consumer actions, such as one-click revocation of data-sharing permissions for that app or company. Easy consumption could imply, for example, prominent posting of a plain-language notice of a recent breach on a company's consumer home page or app sign-in screen for a period after the breach occurred."

These proposals address many of the risks of digital health. At the time of this writing, the debate over this proposed legislation is ongoing with no estimated time for completion or specific driver for action. Concurrently, new digital tools are being introduced daily and the surveillance data market continues to operate and propagate unchecked. We hope that this writing establishes a sense of urgency and builds a strong case for comprehensive action.

Physical security

Beyond the financial and reputational threats of cybercrime, the use of location service by health and other digital apps increases personal security risks. The only safe approach is to understand and assume that active geolocation apps, "see you when you're sleeping and know when you're awake." Activity trackers, vital sign monitoring, even sleep and personal-health-record tools may use, store, or share geolocation data, and users must be attentive and aware due to risks presented by loss of this information and the corresponding personal security issues. For example, technology-enabled violence, abuse, and harassment are on the rise due to the prevalence of stalkerware in the digital ecosystem. One recent National Public Radio survey of domestic violence shelters in the United States found that 85% of domestic violence workers had assisted victims whose abuser tracked them using GPS. The U.S.-based National Network to End Domestic Violence found that 71% of domestic abusers monitor survivors' computer activities, while 54% tracked survivors' cell phones with stalkerware.[19]

To many, these threats may initially sound outlandish, but the warnings coincided with the boom in smartphone use. In 2011, a global information-security nongovernmental organization (NGO), formerly known as the Information Systems Audit and Control Association, now only known as ISACA, published a set of risks that have now been realized. In its report ISACA cautioned, "Problems start to increase when a person's personal information, such as gender, race, occupation and financial history, is combined with information from a GPS and geolocation tags, as the data can be used by criminals to identify an individual's present or future location. This raises the potential of threats ranging from burglary and theft to stalking and kidnapping."[20]

The personal-security profession relies heavily on this type of data to track individuals they are protecting but also uses it to understand possible threat vectors and exposure. According to BlackMoor Technical Services,

> When examining security threats to personnel a key consideration is the predictability of the potential target. If an attacker can predict your location at a given time

in the future, they have no need to invest in costly resources such as physical and electronic surveillance. Essentially, predictable target location greatly simplifies the attack equation. While there are myriad aspects to protecting yourself, your associates, or family members, today we are going to focus on adversary access to personal geolocation data. . . . [Further], [y]our geolocation data can provide a wealth of information about your current and past activities, as well as who you associate with, and is a key factor in developing a personal profile called your "pattern of life."

Geolocation data derived over an extended period of time can provide extremely sensitive and detailed information about a person. Have you visited an oncology center, had appointments with a mental health professional, or visited Planned Parenthood? Anyone with access to your geolocation data knows where you were and will infer what you were doing, or more importantly, what they think you were doing. Obviously, this is a recipe for a privacy disaster, but in terms of personal security, it is also a significant attack enabler.[21]

The value of geolocation data is actually quite high when compared with the relative value of other personal information that can be obtained via cybercrime. As hinted above, geolocation data can actually serve as a unifier for other forms of information, which enables the construction of complex individual patterns of behavior that could not be surmised by other data alone. As the value of data goes up, so does the corresponding level of cyber threat.[22]

As with many aspects of cybersecurity, awareness and personal behavior can play a significant role in lowering risk. Keeping location services disabled or only enabled very selectively is a basic start. In general, anything that improves cyberhygiene will help minimize geolocation threat and should include behavior in healthcare settings, such as using "free" hospital WiFi when visiting healthcare providers. Specific steps also can be taken to examine a phone to see whether it has been jailbroken or contains "stalkerware" apps. Due to the rapid evolution of this technology, we will not share specifics here because they likely will be out of date before this book goes to print. Best practices are to always consult cyberprofessionals at work or via customer support at individual technology providers, given that many recommendations will be device and platform specific.

Medical misinformation

Truly a plague of the digital era, medical misinformation stems from multiple sources. The most benign form of medical misinformation can be simply individuals expressing their own beliefs online or via low-tech means. More malicious forms of medical misinformation include "disinformation," which is disseminated with knowledge that those who succumb to it could be harmed, and "malinformation," which represents a purposeful effort to harm others directly by spreading incorrect information. Regardless of type, medical misinformation may be the most virulent threat of the digital-health era, given that it is responsible for the recurrence of previously eradicated diseases such as measles.

The challenge combatting medical misinformation, especially in democratic countries, is that there are no well-codified or clear dividing lines between what is personal opinion and what is actually misinformation. In the United States, freedom of speech is a given and expected right. That said, running into a crowded building and yelling "fire" clearly will have social and legal consequences, but going onto social media and posting antivaccine information that could just as easily put individuals at risk for serious disease does not (yet) have similar consequences. In an attempt to distinguish misinformation from disinformation and malinformation in the context of possible protective tactics, I published a piece with former U.S. Food and Drug Administration (FDA) Commissioner Rob Califf, MD in the *Journal of the American Medical Association* (*JAMA*) in mid-2019 with an eye toward utilizing cyberdefense strategies to neutralize and prevent medical disinformation and malinformation.[23] The piece quickly proved at least one point, given that I was immediately inundated with hate via e-mail and on social media. The most common criticism being the incorrect claim that I was advocating against free speech. Nothing could be further from the truth.

I suggest the reader seek out the article and enjoy it in its entirety; however, a brief summary follows. The piece starts by citing extensive statistics on medical misinformation and references multiple pleas for help and policy by medical professional organizations and medical journal authors. The approaches suggested to date, however, are not immediately actionable in ways that will address the acute issue. Better science literacy and other educational approaches are essential but not immediately impactful. Similarly, expecting big tech to fix the problem has so far not proven effective, but there is movement on this front that bears watching. In the piece we go on to suggest precise diagnostics and the employment of cyberstrategies. With respect to precise diagnostics, honey pots and other measurement devices can assess Internet signals and aid in determining when information swells are organic, that is, involving disparate opinions of many individuals, or more organized, as in troll armies sponsored by aggressor nation-states. When precise and validated diagnostics point to the latter, we suggest the application of cyberstrategies to nullify the threat. Specifically, we detail the five core cybersecurity functions of the NIST Cybersecurity framework, previously referenced and discussed in the text.

Specifically, it is essential to *identify* and prioritize the most essential health information sources for the public and for practitioners. Equally important is a detailed understanding and quantification of medical misinformation threats. Second, applying the *protect* function to misinformation requires that these trusted and resilient sources of information be adequately safeguarded. Essential healthcare information of the kind intended to inform the public must be protected from damage, destruction, misuse, and corruption, and thus requires a high level of cybersecurity protection. Third, apply the *detect* function, it is necessary to be able to assess and isolate the most harmful forms and vectors of medical misinformation such as *disinformation*, which is disseminated with knowledge that those who succumb to it could be harmed, and *malinformation*, which represents a purposeful effort to harm others directly by spreading incorrect information. Fourth, the *respond* function includes taking appropriate action when a threat incident is detected. Responses can be highly varied and range from defensive responses such as taking critical assets offline to protect them, to offensive options such as a distributed denial of service attack (DDOS) to take down sites that are propagating malinformation on a large scale. This is where cyberattack techniques can be ethically used by law enforcement to contain, counter, disable, and destroy dangerous cyber misinformation attacks. Lastly, the *recover* function focuses on the restoration of any capabilities or services that were impaired by an attack. This should include after-action reviews to (1) ensure full recovery from damaging campaigns, (2) improve protections to meet future threats, and (3) inform comprehensive educational efforts that help the public recognize bogus campaigns.

In addition to these approaches, which are intended to counter disinformation and malinformation, multiple tactics are being employed to deal with misinformation. First, please note that for the purposes of this writing, I am using the term misinformation to refer primarily to the opinions of individuals. Although these opinions can be misguided and equally as destructive to any gullible individual, we must assume that they are honest, in that the believers/speakers/social media posters in question truly believe what they are saying and are only trying to share their opinion.

Starting with tactics being employed by clinicians, some are taking it on themselves to utilize their own time and personal social media accounts to counter misinformation.[24] This can be highly effective but lacks scalability. The primary threat to this approach is trolling by the more organized misinformation movements. I experienced this myself upon publication of the *JAMA* piece that is discussed earlier in this chapter. Shortly after the piece was published, I received dozens of e-mails and a few social media messages claiming that I was calling for censure of free speech. Those who read the article know that I explicitly state that I believe free speech must be protected, and that people are entitled to believe, share, and express their own opinions. The article recommends tactics to deal with large-scale disinformation, which is quite different.

These attacks on my article highlight several key points about the medical misinformation problem. First, there is growing distrust of medicine and science. To me, this is not an information problem. If the public has become so distrusting of institutions that they see conspiracy everywhere and distrust the motives of medical practice, diagnosis, and treatment, then social media posting of these opinions is only a symptom of a much greater problem. The difficulty expands significantly when distrust is layered on top of low scientific literacy. Under the best of conditions, medical communications can be challenging due to complex jargon and unfamiliar situations. A patient may wonder, can the doctor not give me a simple "yes" or "no" answer to my question because they don't know the answer? Are they hedging their bets? Are they just trying to run up my bill? Are they only recommending the vaccine because the pharmaceutical industrial complex is paying them? Given this growing distrust, the use of social media by clinicians to "speak the truth" against misinformation can add to distrust and actually backfire.

We will close out this section with some thoughts from Steven Novella, MD, of Yale University, who published an excellent editorial in *JAMA* in April 2019, wherein he systematically debunks the status quo methodologies that have long been touted as cures for medical misinformation.

> Confronting fraud, pseudoscience, science denial, and misinformation need to be top priorities for the academic, scientific, and medical communities. This must also go beyond just confronting what appears to be a short-term crisis. This is forever. We need a culture change where these priorities are recognized as intrinsic to the scientific enterprise.[25]

Digital bezoar stones and medical charlatanism

We have previously discussed the bezoar stone and the notion of caveat emptor. In many ways, that paradigm is unchanged. Unproven and spurious medical devices predate the modern era of medical product regulation and will likely never fully disappear. There will always be dreamers and charlatans who prey on the hopes of their victims. The technological complexity (Who really knows how their Apple watch works?), the perceived rapid pace of technological advancement and the associated hype, coupled with low scientific literacy and the ever-increasing volume of medical misinformation are all factors that make the patient/consumer more vulnerable to fraud and faulty decision-making.

As I write this from my home, where I am under self-quarantine due to recent high-risk Covid-19 relief work in the rural Southwest, it is far too easy for me to open a Web browser and quickly see quackery and charlatanism. Whether it is the constant debates about the pros and cons of mask wearing, a piece in the *MIT Technology Review* about top-tier health scientists taking a vaccine of their own making, or a fake coronavirus-cure commercial shared by the President of the United States, the toxic mix of misinformation and those looking to profit from selling snake oil is everywhere.[26,27] The single most important thing to understand about this particular toxicity is that it disproportionally affects the most vulnerable patient populations, which why there should be urgent prioritization of systemic countermeasures.[28]

We live in exciting times and many of the promises of digital health are real and worthy of optimism. We must also take care. From CRISPR babies to digital bezoar stones, individuals will always seek their own vision of a healthy life. The medical establishment, as well as medical/scientific social media influencers, must act and tweet responsibly.

Final word on the adversary

Lastly, it is important, once again, to consider the nature of an adversary. Historically, medical adverse events have been studied as accidents, as unintentional harms caused by circumstance or bad luck. The connectivity of the digital world changes that equation by adding the possibility of interference from a bad actor wishing to do harm. Medicine is not yet equipped for this. The concept of the American Medical Association (AMA) vs. the Russian KGB sounds far-fetched, but it is not. It has been proven to be here and now. When medicine adopts digital health technology it inherits a key characteristic of medical misinformation and cyberwarfare, namely, asymmetry. A lone hacker can take down a much more powerful foe because a devastating cyberattack does not require soldiers, extensive resources, or weaponry, but only a computer, technical expertise, and time.

A small number of antivaccine voices have been amplified on the Internet to persuade a large segment of the population to question the entire medical-scientific community, eroding decades of trust in the patient-clinician relationship. The converse aspect of asymmetry is being overpowered by a superior force. Although it is clear that at least some instances of medical misinformation campaigns originate with individual persons, many forms of cyberthreat do not. Until we account for this within product regulation, product use, and healthcare delivery systems, we are leaving ourselves and our most vulnerable to the mercy of those who may have none.

References

1. Jaret P. Exposing Vulnerabilities: How Hackers Could Target Your Medical Devices. *AAMC News*. 2018, November 12. https://www.aamc.org/news-insights/exposing-vulnerabilities-how-hackers-could-target-your-medical-devices
2. Murray K. Healthcare Cyberthreats that Should Keep You Up at Night. Webroot. 2019, October 29. https://www.webroot.com/blog/2019/10/29/healthcare-cyber-threats-that-should-keep-you-up-at-night/
3. Andrews M. The Rise of Medical Identity Theft. *Consumer Reports*. 2016, April https://www.consumerreports.org/medical-identity-theft/medical-identity-theft/
4. Solove D. 10 Reasons Why Privacy Matters. Teachprivacy.com. 2014, January 20. Accessed December 2019. https://teachprivacy.com/10-reasons-privacy-matters/
5. Sterling B. Why Privacy Matters Even If You Have Nothing to Hide. *Wired*. 2011, June 28.
6. Menand L. Why Do We Care So Much About Privacy. *The New Yorker*. 2018, June 11.
7. Greenwald G. Why Privacy Matters. Ted talk. 2014. Accessed December 2019. https://www.ted.com/talks/glenn_greenwald_why_privacy_matters
8. Arne. Why Privacy Matters and Why It Is Time to Fight for It. Tutanota. Accessed December 2019. https://tutanota.com/blog/posts/data-privacy-day/
9. Davis J. 70% of Data in Healthcare Breaches Increases Risk of Fraud. Health IT Security 2019, September 25. Accessed December 2019. https://healthitsecurity.com/news/70-of-data-involved-in-healthcare-breaches-increases-risk-of-fraud
10. Irwin I. How Long Does It Take to Detect a Cyberattack? IT Governance 2019, March 14. Accessed October 2019. https://www.itgovernanceusa.com/blog/how-long-does-it-take-to-detect-a-cyber-attack
11. Garruba T. 5 Ways Health Data Breaches Are Far Worse than Financial Ones. Healthcare IT News. 2014, November 10.
12. Ponemon. 2013 Survey on Medical Identity Theft. September 2013. Downloaded June 2019.
13. Wikipedia. California Privacy Act. Accessed December 2019. https://en.wikipedia.org/wiki/California_Consumer_Privacy_Act
14. Warzel C. Will Congress Ever Pass a Privacy Bill? *New York Times*. 2019. December 10.
15. Shepardson D, and D Bartz. Republican Privacy Bill Would Set US Rules and Preempt California: Senator. Reuters. 2019, December 2.
16. Beckerman M. Americans Will Pay a Price for State Privacy Laws. *New York Times*. 2019, October 14.

17. NCSL. 2019 Consumer Data Privacy Legislation. Ncsl.org. 2020, January 3. Accessed January 2020. http://www.ncsl.org/research/telecommunications-and-information-technology/consumer-data-privacy.aspx

18. Bari L, and DP O'Neill. Rethinking Patient Data Privacy in the Era of Digital Health. *Health Affairs Blog*. 2019, December 12.

19. Shahini A. Smartphones Are Used to Stalk, Control Domestic Abuse Victims. All Things Considered. National Public Radio. 2014, September 15.

20. Info Security Group. ISACA Warns on Mobile Device Geolocation. *Info-Security Magazine*. 2011, September 28. Accessed October 2019 .https://www.infosecurity-magazine.com/news/isaca-warns-on-mobile-device-geo-location/

21. BlackMoor Technical Services. Personal Security. Location, location—geolocation. 2019, April 18. Accessed December 2019. https://blackmoortech.com/f/physical-security-%7C-location-location-geolocation

22. ThreatModeler. The Collateral Damage of a Geolocation Data Breach. 2019, November 13. Accessed December 2019. https://threatmodeler.com/collateral-damage-geolocation-data-breach/

23. Perakslis E, and RM Califf. Employ Cybersecurity Techniques Against the Threat of Medical Misinformation. *JAMA* 2019. 322(3):207–208. doi:10.1001/jama.2019.6857

24. Rubin R. Getting Social: Physicians Can Counteract Misinformation with an Online Presence. *JAMA* 2019. 322(7):598–600. doi:10.1001/jama.2019.10779

25. Armstrong PW, and CD Naylor. Counteracting Health Misinformation: A Role for Medical Journals? *JAMA* 2019. 321(19):1863–1864. doi:10.1001/jama.2019.5168

26. Regalado A. Some Scientists Are Taking a DIY Coronavirus Vaccine, and Nobody Knows If It Is Legal or If It Works. *MIT Technology Review*. 2020, July 29. https://www.technologyreview.com/2020/07/29/1005720/george-church-diy-coronavirus-vaccine/

27. Brito C. Facebook, Twitter and YouTube Take Down False Coronavirus "Cure" Video Shared by Trump. CBS News. 2020, July 28. https://www.cbsnews.com/news/facebook-twitter-youtube-removing-false-covid-19-information-video-trump-share/

28. Freckelton QC I. COVID-19: Fear, Quackery, False Representations and the Law [published online ahead of print, 2020 July 10]. *International Journal of Law and Psychiatry* 2020. 72:101611. doi:10.1016/j.ijlp.2020.101611

10

Nonadversarially Driven Toxicities

Overdiagnosis and overtreatment

One of the most frequently cited consequences of new digital health technologies are overdiagnosis and/or overtreatment. Just as decades of study of incidental renal masses and the utility of mammograms have led to decades of mixed opinion on worthiness of treatment and risk of overtreatment, we must be ready to address the medical validity of a deluge of digital health sensors and tools. Just as in the aforementioned examples, the burden here extends beyond the application of clinician judgment of the digital measure to the increasingly complex clinician–patient dialogue that can result when patients self-monitor and diagnose with complex technologies.

The ability to quantify the potential of overdiagnosis and overtreatment is complicated and limited. One of the more common examples of public health controversies caused by widespread screening of asymptomatic individuals is the prostate-specific antigen (PSA) test in men. The overall impression is that the test leads to overdiagnosis and overtreatment despite the fact that some studies have shown benefit and others have not.[1] Taking the other most commonly discussed and debated model, prophylactic mammograms, the data is even more evolved. A study in Denmark found the screen-detected breast cancer overdiagnosis rates to be between 14.7% and 38.6%.[2] These rates were determined by breast cancer incidence and death rates in several areas of Denmark where screening was introduced at various times in the 1990s. Although the incidence of localized disease increased with the introduction of screening, the incidence of advanced disease did not decrease, indicating overdiagnosis. Interestingly, the previously cited reference, an editorial by the Chief Medical Officer for the American Cancer Society, Dr. Otis Brawley, goes on to debate whether these overdiagnosis rates still represent a public good. Is subjecting 15% to 39% of women to even minor breast care interventions worthwhile if, overall, lives are saved in the process? Truly a great question with many perspectives. For example, in 2016 when a panel of medical experts reiterated its advice from 2009, that mammograms should start at age 50 instead of age 40, and that mammograms be performed every other year versus yearly for certain populations, outrage ensued, especially from patient

Digital Health. Eric D. Perakslis and Martin Stanley, Oxford University Press (2021). © Oxford University Press.
DOI: 10.1093/oso/9780197503133.003.0010

advocacy organizations. Interestingly, the concerns were not immediately focused upon increased health risks for women but rather on concerns that diminishing the perceived necessity of mammograms would lead to poor insurance coverage for vulnerable populations.

Of course, overdiagnosis is not necessarily an issue unless it leads to overtreatment. As a topic, overtreatment is complex. Factors include diagnostic errors, preventative medicine, patient preference and pressure, defensive medicine and fear of malpractice, as well as, generally, medical training.[3] One influential study estimated that 20.6% of overall medical care was unnecessary, including 22.0% of prescription medications, 24.9% of tests, and 11.1% of procedures.[4] Applying these estimates to the cost of health care in the United States reported by the Centers for Medicare & Medicaid Services (CMS), namely some $3.6 trillion, the costs of overtreatment exceed $700 billion annually. Even if these are just ballpark estimates, the impacts are staggering. More importantly, the effects on any given patient cannot be overlooked. Further, from the clinician perspective on overdiagnosis and overtreatment, "Specialists understand how insidious prostate cancer can be. They recognize the problems arising from overdiagnosis and overtreatment, but they also see people suffering from painful metastases or dying from the disease. When you're exposed to that, you're likely going to have a more reserved approach toward surveillance strategies," according to Tudor Borza, MD, MS at the University of Michigan when commenting on trends in prostate cancer detection and treatment in 2017.[5]

When it comes to understanding the potential downsides of overdiagnosis and overtreatment in regard to digital health, the topic is yet to be studied in detail given that digital health tools are just now reaching the market. Let's look at a few examples that are playing out in real time.

Overdiagnosis and overtreatment—Apple Watch case study

Atrial fibrillation (also called AFib or AF) is a quivering or irregular heartbeat (arrhythmia) that can lead to blood clots, stroke, heart failure, and other heart-related complications.[6] According to the Centers for Disease Control and Prevention (CDC), approximately 2% of people younger than age 65 have AFib, while about 9% of people aged 65 years or older have Afib.[7] Standard of care for AFib diagnosis is an electrocardiogram (ECG) or echocardiogram, but because AFib only occurs intermittently in many adults, it may not be found during a brief ECG in clinic and longer-term measurement is needed.

This is often accomplished using Holter monitors, a portable ECG that can record heart events for 24 hours or longer contiguously, or an event recorder, a portable ECG device is intended to monitor your heart activity over a few weeks to a few months. The Apple Watch was cleared for irregular heart rate detection in the fall of 2018. To some, this means that instead of using Holter or event monitors for days or weeks, AFib detection may be available in a consumer device that can be worn 24 hours per day, 365 days per year. This could clearly bring tangible benefit, especially to those who have not been diagnosed with AFib or who are underdiagnosed because they have AFib, but it did not happen to occur during the brief period of time a patient was wearing a Holter or event monitor.

In evaluating the benefits and risks of this new innovation, the first step is to determine the efficacy. Because the device was cleared by the U.S. Food and Drug Administration (FDA) and not approved, we know that it did not undergo full efficacy and safety testing but instead was compared to a predicate device. Early independent studies of efficacy, such as the Apple Heart Study, a massive study of more than 400,000 patients, produced questionable results due to potential patient compliance issues. Specifically, the patients participating wore the Apple Watch and were sent a notification if the smartwatch detected an irregular heartbeat. They were then supposed to follow up with an ECG for verification, but a significant subpopulation did not follow up with the ECG for various reasons. The bottom line was that ECG patches confirmed atrial fibrillation in only 34% of the 450 patients who returned the patches. The remaining, about 66%, had no confirmed atrial fibrillation. During a panel discussion of the trial at the annual meeting of the American College of Cardiology in 2019, Jeanne Poole, professor at the University of Washington in Seattle, said, "This also has the possibility to lead a lot of patients potentially to be treated unnecessarily or prematurely, or flooding doctors' offices and cardiologists' offices with a lot of young people."[8] It should be noted that this study was performed with an older version of the Apple Watch using the heart rate function and not with the newer version, which has the electrocardiogram feature. However, a recent *New England Journal of Medicine* article on this same study stated that the probability of receiving an irregular pulse notification was low. Among participants who received notification of an irregular pulse, 34% had atrial fibrillation on subsequent ECG patch readings, and 84% of notifications were concordant with atrial fibrillation.[9]

Interestingly, both Dr. Poole and the *New England Journal of Medicine* article may be right. In the study, the 84% of notifications that were found to be concordant with AFib represent a subsample of the patient population who were essentially 100% compliant with the highly controlled study protocol. The question is, how often does this happen in real life?

When the potential harms associated with human behaviors are considered the benefit-risk calculus changes. One such instance would be when people who have atrial fibrillation don't consult a doctor about symptoms such as heart palpitations or shortness of breath because they feel falsely reassured by the absence of any alert from their Apple Watch. The new study provides no evidence about the true rate of false negatives in the study population because the researchers did not independently monitor people in whom the device did not detect AFib.[10] Another concern is that a high rate of false positives will send young, healthy people into clinics seeking diagnostics and care. Not only would this add unnecessary cost and burden to the health system, but it also simply could clog the system making it more difficult for the truly infirm to get necessary care. Although this may seem far-fetched, we must consider the fact that smartwatches are not all that common among the older populations who are likely to have AFib, but they are extremely common among the younger and more fit lower-risk population. Like all instances of looking under the lamp post, the fact that most wearers of Apple Watches are younger and more fit should inform us that a high percentage of alerts will result in potential overdiagnosis.

The good news is that these mechanisms of overdiagnosis are not likely to lead to actual overtreatment, but that may depend on how one defines over-treatment. Patients who seek care based upon these notifications are likely to be subjected to confirmatory studies via traditional means, and only in those cases that are confirmed will patients receive medicines or other care. Depending on who you ask, some would consider these confirmatory studies "treatments" in that they require care, incur cost, and require medical over-sight that competes with clinic time for other patients. I tend to fall into this camp, and I personally consider confirmatory studies to be overtreatment if done in excess. This is especially true if the potential risks of the clinical en-vironment are applied to these patients. Others would define care more nar-rowly and would limit it to interventional procedures and/or medicines, but fewer fall into this camp given that confirmatory studies consume resources, cost money, and represent significant utilization of healthcare facilities and professionals.

There are a great many things to study about the Apple Watch and the ECG and irregular heartbeat detection capabilities. It is just as interesting, or even more so, to consider that the actual utility, good or bad, that a healthcare tool offers may be shaped more by market dynamics than by the technical capabilities of the device. In designing digital tools to improve health care, making those tools available to the proper population and enabling or ensuring uptake by those proper populations may be more difficult than developing the device in the first place.

Cyberchondria and stresses on attention and mental health

In addition to the previously discussed challenges of overdiagnosis, the emotional stresses of alarm that unsupervised digital health tools could cause is being shown to be a risk to mental health. Social media use has been definitively linked to depression and self-harm in children and young adults.[11] In addition to depression, social media use has been linked to cell-phone addiction, sleep disturbance, cognitive decline, and shortened attention spans.[12,13] What most of these potential issues have in common is that they increase in severity in aggregate, which should give clinicians pause prior to recommending additional digital interventions. Susceptibility varies across the population.

The term cyberchondria refers to the phenomenon of health anxiety due to consumption of online health information.[14] Hypochondria is a debilitating disorder that occurs in about 1% to 5% of people once in a lifetime.[15] One study of 471 people in Germany found that participants with symptoms of hypochondria used the Internet more frequently for health-related purposes and also frequented more online services than individuals without symptoms. Most online health services were rated as more reliable by individuals with symptoms of hypochondria. Changes to behavior such as doctor hopping or ordering nonprescribed medicine online were considered more likely by individuals with symptoms of hypochondria. It should be noted, however, that the methods of recruiting for this study, via various health websites, provided an already enriched population given that the initial sampling was found to have almost 25% hypochondriacs versus the percentage normally found in the population of roughly 5%. This is an important point with respect to digital health advertising and hype in that the populations that are most likely to be encountered using these sites are already highly inclined toward hypochondria and distrust of clinical medicine, making them more vulnerable.

The effects of Internet use on hypochondria have been documented for more than 20 years. "For hypochondriacs, the Internet has absolutely changed things for the worse," says Brian Fallon, MD, professor of psychiatry at Columbia University and the coauthor of *Phantom Illness: Recognizing,*

Understanding and Overcoming Hypochondria (1996).[16] The core basis of hypochondria, and now cyberchondria, is the obsession with symptoms and the relentless search for resolution and, at times, validation. The increasingly available range of consumer-grade digital health tools are very likely to increase this phenomenon. "Illness often becomes a central part of a hypochondriac's identity," says Arthur Barsky, MD, of Harvard Medical School and the author of *Worried Sick: Our Troubled Quest for Wellness* (1988).[17] As a result, a hypochondriac's work and relationships suffer. And those with the condition aren't the only ones who pay the price: According to Fallon, hypochondria costs billions of dollars a year in unnecessary medical tests and treatments. "What hypochondriacs have trouble accepting is that normal, healthy people have symptoms," says Barsky. Hypochondriacs tend to be very aware of bodily sensations that most people live with and ignore. To a hypochondriac, an upset stomach becomes a sign of cancer and a headache can only mean a brain tumor. The stress that goes along with this worry can make the symptoms even worse. Digging into the specifics of self-diagnosis via the Internet, the two most likely diagnoses are anxiety and depression, further suggesting the increased susceptibility of emotional health to the Internet and digital tools.

Another vulnerable subpopulation appears to be health students. In one study at Ege University in Turkey, the cyberchondria scores of students with health problems are higher in the whole scale and in "distress and mistrust of medical professional" subscales. As the frequency of scanning on the Internet increases, the scores of cyberchondria also increase significantly. Medical students had significantly higher scores in "distress, excessiveness, and reassurance" subscales. Male students' "mistrust of medical professional and compulsion" subscale scores were also higher. It was determined that the presence of the health problem affected the cyberchondria.[18] The interesting element of this study is that increased use of digital data outside of traditional clinical interaction inevitably increases distrust of the system. Further, this distrust then increases susceptibility to misinformation, which often can be spread by disaffected medical professionals.

Some have gone so far as to say that "everyone who gets into the world of digital health will become a cyberchondriac to a certain extent. So, the real question is not how to avoid becoming a cyberchondriac, as we'll all get into it, but how we can overcome anxiety as fast as possible and use our newfound knowledge for something good."[19] Although this is clearly an overstatement, it is rare in that this author is calling out the inevitability of the risks of cyberchondria proactively and suggesting solutions. This is a stark but positive contrast to the flood of digital health hype that is far more likely to tout unproven benefits and completely ignore the possibility of accompanying downsides. The piece goes on to make several common-sense suggestions to avoid cyberchondria that actually may be quite useful for clinicians. Instead of telling patients, and one another, that they should not search the Internet, self-diagnose, or "trust Google," the following may provide a better basis for communication: **"Recognize that the Internet is a double-edged sword."**

"It could be incredibly helpful in finding doctors or communities, but it could also give you a very misleading picture if you try to self-diagnose. So be informed, track your health, note the changes, learn about our 'Ask Me About Digital' badge campaign to get information on how to use technologies to your advantage. Importantly, don't leave out your doctor, be a partner, let's figure it out together."[20] Truly solid advice, which recommends the use of confirmation sources as an effective defense against misinformation.

Financial toxicity

The digital health industry and its investors are extremely fond of touting explosive market opportunities, as in, "Digital health market is expected to reach $379B, representing to register a CAGR (compound annual growth rate) of 26% over 2017–2024."[21] But who is expected to pay the price? At a time when financial distress has become a calculable patient-reported outcome, it is also being reported as more severe than physical, family, and emotional distress by advanced-cancer patients.[22,23] Unless sensible care is taken, potentially expensive and nonreimbursable digital tools will only muddy the value waters. Further, one of the risks of financial toxicity is that it can occur as a cascading impact. For example, patients may seek care from multiple sources concurrently or sequentially as a result of overdiagnosis, and this behavior can lead to even more diagnostic tests or treatment.

But are digital tools and the resulting data potentially part of the solution? Given the time spent on electronic medical records by care providers, and given the fact that these systems are truly billing aggregators at the core, it would make sense that cost information be included, but it is not. Clinicians typically can see treatment options but not cost information and therefore are "blind and clueless to the cost of care."[24] One would think that this was easily fixed but, as we have discussed, flexibility is far from the nature of most commercial electronic health records. Another frequently touted cost-reducing digital innovation is telehealth. One study of telehealth at Philadelphia-based Jefferson Healthcare found that the net cost savings to the patient or payer per telemedicine visit of $19 to $121 represented a meaningful cost savings when compared with the

$49 cost of an on-demand visit. The primary source of the generated savings is from avoidance of the emergency department, because it is by far the most expensive of the alternative care options provided.[25] In rural settings the total cost savings, including travel time, missed time from work, travel expenses, etc., are likely even higher. A 1998–2002 study of the Rural Hospital Program in Arkansas determined that without telemedicine, 94% of patients would travel more than 70 miles for medical care; 84% would miss one day of work; and 74% would spend $75–$150 for additional family expenses. With telemedicine, 92% of patients saved $32 in fuel costs; 84% saved $100 in wages; and 74% saved $75–$150 in family expenses.[26] Further, a University of Iowa study showed that patients were seen six times more quickly at rural hospitals using telemedicine in their emergency departments than in those without.[27] These benefits concur with the promise that digital tools will make remote care more effective and available.

Moving from brief episodic healthcare needs into the more complex chronic disease space, mHealth and remote digital tools are starting to demonstrate financial benefits for patients. One study of chronic diabetes management found that patients using digital health tools that include wireless devices and a telehealth link to their care providers can cut about 22%, approximately $80, of their monthly medical expenses through better care management. Those reduced costs also translate to better long-term health outcomes and more efficiency in the doctor's office.[28] In many ways, this may be the greatest economic opportunity for digital health, given that so much of our healthcare expenditures are utilized to manage chronic care. Specifically, according to a 2018 Milken Institute report, when lost economic productivity is included, the total economic impact was $3.7 trillion. This is equivalent to nearly 20% of the U.S. gross domestic product.[29] Stunning.

One objection raised by telehealth skeptics is that visits could cost more over the longer term because of the need for excessive follow-up with in-person appointments. A Humana study of this very issue, however, determined comparable rates of follow-up visits between telemedicine and in-office visits within two weeks. At the same time, telemedicine had slightly higher numbers for physician (6.6%), emergency department (1.3%), and urgent care referrals (0.9%) compared to in-office visits for those referrals (5.1%, 1.1%, and 0.1%, respectively).[30] The numbers make sense given that there will always be significant limitations on the types of clinical observations that can be made via video versus in-person visits. Interestingly, another often-cited concern of telehealth is the loss of continuity of care, somewhat the opposite of the concern that telehealth will lead to excessive follow ups. Further,

telehealth does rely on expensive equipment at the clinical site and the availability of adequate internet bandwidth connectivity at the patient home; in
fact, many patients may not have broadband.[31]

Given the risks and ability to raise healthcare costs via overused technology,
overdiagnosis, and overtreatment, together with the potential to lower healthcare costs by virtualization and remote access, the economics of digital health
are an excellent study in healthcare benefit-risk. Like many things in healthcare efficiency and quality, it may actually be the payers who perform the detailed study and experimentation that will be required to maintain a positive
balance for patients.

Medical device deregulation

Although laudable in intent, recent moves by the U.S. FDA to enable innovation in medical devices are cause for concern with respect to medical device
evaluation and approval. In particular, there are significant concerns about
the FDA Pre-Cert program. First, there are questions on this type of regulatory approach, such as where it has been done before, and whether it has been
demonstrated as an effective means of regulation.[32] Probably the most compelling criticism of the Pre-Cert program has come from the global medical
device industry itself. Specifically, there have been multiple calls from medical
device manufacturers and experts for the FDA to consider utilizing preexisting and well-codified benefit-risk frameworks, such as those established by
the International Medical Device Regulators Forum (IMDRF), which enable
a comprehensive and global approach to medical device benefit risk.[33] Indeed,
the IMDRF frameworks for the clinical evaluation of Software as a medical
device (SaMD) products and for risk characterization of these products are
truly excellent and comprehensive and should be given serious consideration.
Otherwise, the United States is simply dropping safety standards without evidence to support patient safety concerns.

The results are clear. Although the FDA likes to tout metrics of devices
approved, or exempted from the approval process, as signs of innovation
and patient care, these numbers ring hollow in the absence of equally valid
corresponding safety and quality statistics. For example, in 2003 the FDA
announced eight Class 1 device recalls, which are defined as recalls in which
there is a "reasonable probability" that a device will "cause serious adverse
health consequences or death." In 2016, by contrast, there were 117 Class 1
device recalls, affecting hundreds of thousands of patients.[34] The challenge is
compounded by what some feel is intentional obfuscation of medical device

safety reporting by the FDA. There have been multiple reports of hidden medical device safety databases that are utilized for decision-making but are not publicly available. One study by the International Consortium of Investigative Journalists (ICIJ) showed that the FDA provided such exemptions to breast implant manufacturers, with the result that tens of thousands of reports have been submitted privately and are not reflected in the Manufacturer and End User Facility Device Experience (MAUDE) database. ICIJ alleges that the 350,000 reports related to breast implants received by the FDA since 2009 represent more than 20 times the number that are publicly available through the MAUDE database.[35] Another study by the Kaiser Health Network, published in March 2019, further explored the alternative summary reporting system, noting its obfuscating effect on the safety statistics of surgical staplers. The report found an astonishing discrepancy between public and private reporting of surgical staplers dangerously misfiring or having other malfunctions.

In another unprecedented instance, the FDA has gone as far as declaring the benefits of unregulated digital tools outweigh the risks. According to the FDA's *Report on Non-Device Software Functions: Impact to Health and Best Practices—December 2018*, unregulated digital health tools improve clinical outcomes, promote physical activity and weight loss, increase behavior that would lead to greater medication adherence, provide evidence of better self-management of chronic conditions, and reduce patient safety events or medication errors.[36] Although these statements are fine when thought of in a general sense, speaking to potential issues of safety in a general sense is not what the FDA has ever done in the past. For example, we are not likely to see similar quotes declaring that, "in general, drugs are good for sick people," yet we are seeing such statements, backed by very little or no data, regarding medical devices. Again, the statement that most digital health apps are beneficial because they bring a sense of awareness to health that often benefits users is not incorrect, but it is also not harmless, because it doesn't account for the accompanying tradeoffs or downsides, which we have highlighted. In fact, studies have shown the opposite, namely, that most health apps offer little benefit.

One influential study in *Nature Digital Medicine* on whether smartphone popularity and *m*Health apps provide a huge potential to improve health outcomes for millions of patients. The researchers wrote, "We found only a small fraction of the available *m*Health apps had been tested and the body of evidence was of very low quality. Our recommendations for improving the quality of evidence and reducing research waste and potential harm in this nascent field include encouraging app effectiveness testing prior to release, designing less biased trials, and conducting better reviews with robust risk of bias assessments."[37] Beyond the contradictory findings by the FDA that these apps are "generally beneficial," the FDA guidance also implies that these apps are all of similar quality and reliability, which is also untrue. Even a large federal agency such as the FDA must not be tone deaf to the dichotomy arising between innovation and patient safety. Certainly, generalizations that communicate the benefits of entire classes of products that have not been tested individually, or at least statistically sampled, is a practice likely to cause harm and to encourage questionable actors.

Going forward, the greatest concern with medical device regulation is likely to be algorithms, as we discuss in the chapter on artificial intelligence (AI). The initial approaches to algorithm regulation by the FDA have been to more or less treat algorithms as software and utilize quality software engineering practices to ensure accuracy and safety. This falls short for multiple reasons. First, advanced algorithms are not simply software; they learn, they forecast, they correlate, and they predict. Equating algorithms with software would be analogous to reviewing the statistical database for a drug clinical and saying that as long as the statistical software was well-maintained by qualified personnel, the database must be valid regardless of whether the programmed math was accurate. Instead of classifying algorithms as software, regulators must dig in and study the complexities and potential side effects of these immensely complex tools to ensure that their performance is measurable and explainable when put into practice.

Although not completely understood, certain types of risks associated with using AI have become clear. At the top of the list is the "black box" problem, which refers to AI explain ability. Most users simply do not understand how an algorithm arrives at an answer. In medicine, where the scientific underpinnings of even the most complex procedures must be fully understood by those who prescribe and utilize them, this causes real problems. First, this creates a lack of trust. Clinicians will rightfully struggle with the ethics, and resulting liabilities, of utilizing tools they don't and can't fully understand. The second issue involves the context of reliability. It is known that algorithms can have extremely context-specific bias built in due to their design and the nature of training data used. The resulting error could be that an algorithm that performed in a certain manner in one institution, where it was trained, could perform very differently in another institution based upon specific practices, data definitions, or policies at the training institution. Even simple subtleties in vernacular could contribute to hidden bias. The third— and recently very high-profile—risk associated with algorithms is hidden bias caused by limited training sets. Most notably, a study published in *Science* in October 2019 found that an algorithm widely used in U.S. hospitals to allocate health care to patients has been systematically discriminating against black people.[38] Specifically, the study concluded that the algorithm was less likely to refer black people than white people who were equally sick to programs that aim to improve care for patients with complex medical needs. Hospitals and insurers use the algorithm and others like it to help manage care for about 200 million people in the United States each year.

Lastly, these types of bias are especially troubling as public health concerns because (1) the producers of the tools may not even be aware of the bias in their machine, and (2) most such tools are considered confidential intellectual property (IP) and are not open to outside study. Indeed, this may be the greatest argument for stronger regulation by the FDA of these tools, wherein an impartial third party is required to study them in a manner that does not expose important IP. IP is similarly protected in the drug review and approval process.

Medical and/or user error

As previously discussed, medical errors are a significant source of death and disability in the United States. When evaluating the safety of medical drugs and devices, the context of use and the level and type of supervision are highly relevant. Just as the dispensing of certain drugs is only allowed by prescription, which requires physician supervision, digital health tools can be quite dangerous in unskilled hands. This paradigm is further complicated in digital health where, unlike the mechanism of action of a familiar drug, the prescribing clinician may have no idea how a specific device works or how to diagnose or correct malfunctions. Just as great care has been taken by the medical community around closed-loop glycemic control due to the high risk of causing insulin administration errors, digital health tools must be carefully evaluated as causes of inadvertent self-harm.

Public opinion on the current safety status quo with medical devices is consistent with the call for change. Whether it is Congress sending pointed letters to the FDA requesting evidence that the Pre-Cert program is safe for digital tools, or whether it is the public outrage following a global investigation that has found that unsafe medical devices have caused 1.7 million injuries globally and almost 83,000 deaths in the last 12 years, the public wants answers and solutions to this important issue.[39] According to the Patient Safety Network of the U.S. Agency for Healthcare Research and Quality, "Medical device-associated errors are common, costly, and often cause preventable harm. A 2008 estimate indicates the annual cost of medical errors to be $17.1 billion to the United States economy, with device-associated errors among the top 10 contributors to this number."[40] A systematic review found that more than 23% of errors in the operating room involve device-related issues. A substantial proportion of device-related errors are user errors that occur due to unintended or unanticipated interactions between devices and users in complex work environments. Evidence indicates that medical device-use errors may be more frequent and cause more harm than device failures (e.g., malfunctions).

Given the prevalence of harm from improper and/or accidental medical device use, it is essential that risks be evaluated to the underlying root causes. According to Conrad Stolz from *24x7* magazine,

> Root Cause Analysis (RCA) methods are based on a recognition that the immediate (proximate) cause of an adverse event is usually not the root (fundamental) cause. The RCA process is essentially a series of "why" questions that are repeated until one or more root causes is identified. Why did the patient receive an overdose of medication through the infusion pump? Why was the pump set up incorrectly? Why was the nurse unfamiliar with the pump? Why is the pump so difficult to use? Why did the hospital select that pump? Only when we get to the root of the matter can we begin to develop responses that are likely to be successful.[41]

Taking these questions to the home setting where digital tools will be utilized in medically unsupervised ways, it is clear that many of these questions would be difficult to answer and that great care should be taken when placing complex technologies into the home environment.

If we can assume that user errors can be minimized via proper training and supervision, and we actually have little choice but to accept these things as true despite the obvious flaws, we must then consider and acknowledge the additional vulnerabilities of these devices themselves. Using one of the oldest and best-understood examples of technology-enabled chronic disease management, diabetes, we have seen most possible concerns realized. Specifically, we have seen that these devices can be tampered with and disabled via intent or accident. As reported by *Wired* in July of 2019 by Lily Hay Newman,

> . . .two cyber security researchers, Billy Rios and Jonathan Butts discovered disturbing vulnerabilities in Medtronic's popular MiniMed and MiniMed Paradigm insulin pump lines. An attacker could remotely target these pumps to withhold insulin from patients, or to trigger a potentially lethal overdose. And yet months of negotiations with Medtronic and regulators to implement a fix proved fruitless. So the researchers resorted to drastic measures. They built an Android app that could use the flaws to kill people. Rios and Butts, who work at the security firm QED

Security Solutions, had first raised awareness about the issue in August 2018 with a widely publicized talk at the Black Hat security conference in Las Vegas. Alongside that presentation, the Food and Drug Administration and Department of Homeland Security warned affected customers about the vulnerabilities as did Medtronic itself. But no one presented a plan to fix or replace the devices. To spur a full replacement program, which ultimately went into effect at the end of June, Rios and Butts wanted to convey the true extent of the threat.[42,43]

To the authors, this remains the key unmet issue in digital health, that vulnerabilities and risks are being exposed in well-documented and credible fashion, but it is not affecting regulatory strategy in any way. Further, what good do FDA warnings do for the average citizen? What are concerned patients expected to do? Ask their doctors? Sure, they can do that but what are doctors supposed to do? All they really can do is reference back to the FDA, a federal agency that approves these devices as low risk but then issues unactionable public warnings.

Digital dependency case study: The Dexcom outage

Unlike the Medtronic vulnerability, which was proactively discovered and ameliorated, diabetes patients and caregivers have recently experienced outages of applications that they consider critical to life-preserving care. Around 1 AM Eastern Standard Time on November 30 through the early morning hours of December 2, the Dexcom Follow app stopped working for more than 48 hours. According to the mother of an affected patient writing in the diabetes magazine *A Sweet Life,*

> . . . the outage made me realize how dependent I've become on being able to see our daughter's blood glucose number all the time—how reliant I am on using Follow as a safety net. And how vulnerable I feel when that safety net is gone. (Our daughter, Bisi, was diagnosed when she was six, in 2012. First, she started using a pump; then, in 2014, the Dexcom CGM; we started being able to see her glucose number on our phones the following year.) Judging by the 5,500 (and counting) comments on Dexcom's Facebook page in response to the outage, many people felt the same way I did. The Follow app has become an integral part of how we help Bisi manage diabetes. We rely on it particularly at night, to alert us and wake us up if Bisi's blood sugar has gone too low or too high. But, really, we rely on it 24 hours a day, because it helps give us peace of mind as Bisi spends more and more time without us—at the park; walking to the movie theater; playing sports; hanging out at friends' house.[44]

Dexcom blamed the outage, and associated impact to availability, on an overloaded server.[45] That digital health inherits common IT issues, some would say is unavoidable, that these result in an incident that can keep thousands of users from accessing critical blood sugar data feels irresponsible.

The ever-increasing infatuation and/or addiction to things digital has been referred to as digital dependency.[46] Descriptions of the symptomology of the phenomenon are fascinating and disturbing. According to *Psychology Today,* nomophobia, the fear of being without a mobile device, or beyond mobile phone contact, is increasing rapidly.[47] One of the more comprehensive descriptions of digital dependency comes from Ofcom, the regulator of communications services in the United Kingdom (UK). Ofcom's Communication Market Report, published in August of 2018, provides significant insight. According to the report, in the UK,

> ...17% of people owned a smartphone a decade ago. That has now reached 78%, and 95% among those aged 16–24 years. The smartphone is now the device people say they would miss the most, dominating many people's lives in both positive and negative ways. People in the UK now check their smartphones, on average, every 12 minutes of the waking day. Two in five adults (40%) first look at their phone within five minutes of waking up, climbing to 65% of those aged under 35. Similarly, 37% of adults check their phones five minutes before lights out, again rising to 60% of users under 35 years of age.[48]

Further, it is clear that the dependency on digital devices is not tempered by caution or even compliance with respect to corresponding risks. In fact, many have become so dependent on convenience that most ignore warnings. Specifically, it has been reported that between 87% and 92% of public Wi-Fi users ignore security warnings, that 41% of users cannot tell the difference between secure and unsecured Wi-Fi networks, and that 57% of survey respondents said they can't wait more than a few minutes before logging onto a Wi-Fi network or asking for the password after arriving at a café, hotel, or friend's home.[49,50,51] Further, most users, 88%, use their cell phone while driving and share account passwords despite organized campaigns and constant reminders to the contrary.[52,53] The security industry refers to these specific issues and barriers as habituation and research has shown that the more individuals are exposed to certain types of warnings, the more they will ignore them.[54]

The Dexcom outage is a warning that digital dependency and associated behaviors appear to have changed the practices of some parents. Prior to continuous glucose monitoring tools such as the Dexcom CGM, parents often felt the need to set alarms throughout the day and night to remind them to monitor blood sugar. CGM tools represent a significant benefit, but how much should we depend upon them? Are they life support or convenience? Do manufacturers, users, and regulators truly understand the difference?

The Dexcom product information website is no better or worse than the typical medical device site. Along with a significant amount of advertising, there are multiple FAQs and long lists of safety precautions shown but not on the same pages as the advertising.[55,56,57] Missing from these pages are clearly described best practices and patterns of use that will help proactively ensure proper use and realistic expectations for users. From the scale of the outrage exhibited toward Dexcom on social media following their outage, it is clear that thousands of families felt that the tools provided life support, even though Dexcom clearly has never promised anything other than convenience.[58] Properly unpacking the complexities here requires deep interrogation, not only of our dependency on technologies and the resulting habituation, but also of our own behaviors and expectations as developers, prescribers, and users.

First, we must expect that patients and caregivers are unlikely to use the tools "as directed." The expectation of user behavior may be more accurately characterized as hazardous rather than diligent. Back in my days of repairing home health equipment, one of the most frequent items that came across my bench were oxygen concentrators, medical devices that concentrated the oxygen from room air via a molecular sieve process based upon rapid pressure swing absorption. These devices were primarily prescribed for patients with COPD and other respiratory illnesses. Despite the hazards of highly concentrated oxygen being clearly labeled on the devices, at least half of them would return from the field with visible cigarette burns on the casings.

Second, knowledge is quickly lost if not kept fresh, current, and available. Beyond the issue of recklessness, many of the safety consequences of device misuse are caused by operator error and/or ignorance. During that time 30 years ago, another of my projects was to test, inspect, and verify the operation of monitors designed to warn parents of the likelihood of sudden infant death syndrome in their infants. Back then the risks of device misuse, in particular the potential choking hazards for infants if they became entangled in the device leads while sleeping or moving about in a crib were well-known and rigorously instilled into parents by visiting nurses. Yet, decades later, the risks for infants sleeping with device cords continue to result in catastrophe and, unlike back then, analogous pediatric monitoring devices are available online and without prescription.[59,60]

Third, the benefits and risks of digital health technologies must be objectively accessed and communicated to all parties. The limitations and inadequacies of typical end user license agreements are well known but the potential harms are not well documented.[61] Further, generic statements and reports from regulators that claim the benefits of unregulated digital health tools outweigh the potential risks are a disservice to the public as (1) general information is not that useful to parents or patients when they are deciding whether to try tool X or tool Y; and (2) the credibility of these statements is not based in or substantiated by randomized clinical trials and is still the topic of active debate.[62,63] Fourth, we must understand and account for the fact that digital health tools seldom exist in a vacuum but rather in an highly complex and ever-changing coexistence with an almost infinite number of possible other apps and systems that amplify risk.

Moving forward, human nature must be embedded within digital health tool delivery and management strategies. The solution framework must include education, advocacy, legislation, and regulation to ensure the privacy and security of a public that simply does not understand the risks they are taking, the threats posed, or the way in which their data are being used.[64] Training on digital health tools must be comprehensive and include basic digital hygiene, as well as detailed scenario planning for outages, disruptions, and malfunctions. Digital health tools must incorporate and train redundancy scenarios.

Lastly, would any of this have prevented the Dexcom outage? No, but it may have greatly lessened the emotional and medical impacts of the outage and that is the primary purpose of risk management. Dexcom failed to communicate, but if the outage was Internet-caused, no one would have heard them if they tried.

References

1. Harvard Health Publishing. The Pros and Cons of PSA Screening. Harvard Medical School. Accessed November 2019. https://www.health.harvard.edu/healthbeat/the-pros-and-cons-of-psa-screening
2. Brawley OW. Accepting the Existence of Breast Cancer Overdiagnosis. *Annals of Internal Medicine* 2017. 166(5):364–365. doi:10.7326/M16-2850
3. Advisory.com staff. What's Behind the Epidemic of Overtreatment? Blame Medical Training. Advisory.com. 2019, April 30.
4. Lyu H et al. Overtreatment in the United States. *PloS One* 2017. 12(9):e0181970. doi:10.1371/journal.pone.0181970
5. Fawcett N. Prostate Cancer Treatment Rates Drop, Reflecting Changes in Screening Recommendations. *University of Michigan Health Blog.* 2017, January 9.

6. American Heart Association. What is Atrial Fibrillation? Heart.org. Accessed December 2019.https://www.heart.org/en/health-topics/atrial-fibrillation/what-is-atrial-fibrillation-afib-or-af

7. CDC. *Atrial Fibrillation*. Accessed December 2019. https://www.cdc.gov/dhdsp/data_statistics/fact_sheets/fs_atrial_fibrillation.htm

8. Terry M. Apple Watch Atrial Fibrillation Study has High Rate of False Positives. *BioSpace*. 2019, March 18.

9. Perez MV et al. Large-Scale Assessment of a Smartwatch to Identify Atrial Fibrillation. *New England Journal of Medicine* 2019. 381(20):1909–1917.

10. Huston L. Beware the Hype Over the Apple Watch Heart App. The Device Could Do More Harm than Good. *STAT*. 2019, March 15.

11. Shafi RMA, PA Nakonezny, M Romanowicz, AL Nandakumar, L Suarez, and PE Croarkin. The Differential Impact of Social Media Use on Middle and High School Students: A Retrospective Study. *Journal of Child and Adolescent Psychopharmacology* 2019. 29(10):746–752.

12. De-Sola Gutiérrez J, F Rodríguez de Fonseca, and G Rubio. Cell-Phone Addiction: A Review. *Front Psychiatry* 2016. 7:175.

13. Makin S. Searching for Digital Technology's Effects on Well-Being. *Nature*. 2018, November 28.

14. Eichenberg C, and M Schott. Use of Web-Based Health Services in Individuals With and Without Symptoms of Hypochondria: Survey Study. *Journal of Medical Internet Research* 2019. 21.

15. Leigh H, and J Streltzer. *Handbook of Consultation-Liaison Psychiatry*. Cham: Springer, 2015.

16. WebMD. Internet Makes Hypochondria Worse. *WebMD*. Accessed December 2019. https://www.webmd.com/balance/features/internet-makes-hypochondria-worse#1

17. Barsky AJ. *Worried Sick: Our Troubled Quest for Wellness*. Little Brown & Co., 1988.

18. Bati AH, A Mandiracioglu, F Govsa, and O Çam. Health Anxiety and Cyberchondria among Ege University Health Science Students. *Nurse Education Today* 2018. 71:169–173.

19. Medical Futurist. How to Overcome Being a Cyberchondriac? *Medical Futurist*. 2018, August 30.

20. Medical Futurist. Ask Me About My Digital Badge. *TMF*. 2018, June 26.

21. Pennic F. Report: Digital Health Market to Reach $379 Billion by 2024. *Global Market Insights*. 2018, June 18.

22. de Souza JA et al. Measuring Financial Toxicity as a Clinically Relevant Patient-Reported Outcome: The Validation of the Comprehensive Score for Financial Toxicity (COST). *Cancer* 2017. 123(3):476–484.

23. Delgado-Guay M et al. Financial Distress and Its Associations With Physical and Emotional Symptoms and Quality of Life Among Advanced Cancer Patients. *Oncologist* 2015. 20(9):1092–1098.

24. O' Donnell W. Ease Financial Toxicity by Putting Electronic Medical Records to Work. *STAT* 2019, September 16.

25. Cheney C. Cost Savings for Telemedicine Estimated at $19 to $120 Per Patient Visit. *Health Leaders*. 2019, May 7. Accessed December 2019. https://www.healthleadersmedia.com/clinical-care/cost-savings-telemedicine-estimated-19-120-patient-visit

26. Bynum AB, CA Irwin, CO Cranford, and GS Denny. The Impact of Telemedicine on Patients' Cost Savings: Some Preliminary Findings. *Telemedicine Journal and E-Health* 2003. 9(4):361–367.

27. Mohr NM et al. Emergency Department Telemedicine Shortens Rural Time-To-Provider and Emergency Department Transfer Times. *Telemedicine Journal and E-Health* 2018. 24(8):582–593.

28. Whaley CM et al. Reduced Medical Spending Associated with Increased Use of a Remote Diabetes Management Program and Lower Mean Blood Glucose Values. *Journal of Medical Economics* 2019. 22(9):869–877.

29. Waters H, and M Graf. Chronic Diseases Are Taxing Our Healthcare System and Economy. *STAT*. 2018, May 31.

30. Pifer M. Humana Study Touts Telehealth Cost Cuts with Comparable Follow Ups. *Healthcare Dive*. 2018, July 18.

31. eVisit. 10 Pros and Cons of Telemedicine. Evisit.com. 2018, May 25. Accessed December 2019. https://evisit.com/resources/10-pros-and-cons-of-telemedicine/

32. Mezher M. Senators Reiterate Concern About FDA's Software Pre-Cert Program. Raps.org. 2019, October 30. Accessed December 2019.

33. IMDRF. Recognized Standards. Accessed December 2019. http://www.imdrf.org/workitems/wi-imdrfstandards.asp

34. Joshi A et al. Trends in Medical Device Recalls. Medtechintelligence.com. 2019, May 21.

35. https://www.medicaldevice-network.com/features/medical-device-safety/

36. U.S. FDA. Report on Non-Device Software Functions: Impact to Health and Best Practices. 2018, December.

37. Byambasuren O, S Sanders, E Beller, and P Glasziou. Prescribable *m*Health Apps Identified from an Overview of Systematic Reviews. *NPJ Digital Medicine* 2018. 1:12.

38. Obermeyer, Z., B Powers, C Vogeli, and S Mullainathan. *Science* 2019. 336: 447–453.

40. Healthcare It News. Unsafe Medical Devices Allowed into Global Markets Harm Patients, Investigation Reveals. 2018, December 4. Accessed December 2019. https://www.healthcareitnews.com/news/unsafe-medical-devices-allowed-global-markets-harm-patients-investigation-reveals

41. Gurses AP, and P Doyle. Medical Devices in the "Wild." *Patient Safety Network*. 2014, December. Accessed December 2019. https://psnet.ahrq.gov/web-mm/medical-devices-wild

42. Stolze C. Six Things We Can Do About Medical Device User Errors. *24x7*. 2007, January 31. Accessed December 2019. https://www.24x7mag.com/standards/safety/medical-device-errors/six-things-we-can-do-about-medical-device-user-errors/

43. Hay-Newman L. These Hackers Made an App that Kills to Prove a Point. *Wired*. 2019, July 16.

44. Bacon K. The Dexcom Follow App Crash and the Ensuing Outrage. *A Sweet Life*. 2019, December. Accessed December 2019. https://asweetlife.org/the-dexcom-follow-app-crash-and-the-ensuing-outrage/

45. Farr C. Dexcom Glitch Kept Parents of Children with Diabetes in the Dark Over Their Conditions This Weekend. *CNBC*. 2019, December 2.

46. Kumar S. Our Digital Dependency. *Mathrubhumi*. 2018, April 1.

47. Elmore T. Nomophobia. A Rising Trend in Students. *Psychology Today*. 2014, September 18.

48. Ofcom. A Decade of Digital Dependency. 2018, August 2. Accessed December 2019. https://www.ofcom.org.uk/about-ofcom/latest/features-and-news/decade-of-digital-dependency

49. VPN Geeks. 5 Frightening Statistics That Mean IT's Time to Move to a Mobile VPN. Vpngeeks.com. Accessed January 2020. https://www.vpngeeks.com/mobile-vpn/

50. Sophos. Why People Ignore Security Alerts Up to 87% of the Time. *Naked Security*. 2016, August 19. Accessed December 2019. https://nakedsecurity.sophos.com/2016/08/19/why-people-ignore-security-alerts-up-to-87-of-the-time/

51. Symantec. 2017 Norton Wi-Fi Risk Report. Nortonlifelock.com. Accessed December 2019. https://www.nortonlifelock.com/about/newsroom/press-kits/norton-wifi-risk-report-2017

52. Deyan G. 61+ Revealing Smart Phone Statistics for 2020. *TechJury*. 2019, March 28.

53. Yakowicz W. Study Finds 95% of People Share Up to 6 Passwords. *Inc*. 2016, February 18.

54. Alhadeff A, and A Blau. The Problem With Your Computer's Security Warnings. Ideas42. Accessed December 2019. https://www.ideas42.org/blog/problem-computers-security-warnings/

55. Dexcom.com. What Is Continuous Glucose Monitoring (CGM)? Accessed January 2020. https://www.dexcom.com/continuous-glucose-monitoring

56. Dexcom.com. Dexcom G6 CGM System FAQ. Accessed January 2020. https://www.dexcom.com/faq/g6

57. Dexcom.com. Safety Information. Accessed January 2020. https://www.dexcom.com/safety-information

58. Parmar A. Dexcom's IT Outage Shows Fabulous Device Maker Floundering with Patient Communication. *MedCity News*. 2019, December 4.

59. CPSC Blogger. Baby Monitor Cords Have Strangled Children. Onsafety.cpsc.gov 2011, February 11. Accessed January 2020. https://onsafety.cpsc.gov/blog/2011/02/11/baby-monitor-cords-have-strangled-children/

60. Bruce-Watt E. Grieving Mom's Warning after Baby is Strangled to Death by Baby Monitor Cord. *New York Post*. 2019, March 26.

61. Newitz A. Dangerous Terms: A User's Guide to EULAs. Eff.org. 2005, February. Accessed January 2020. https://www.eff.org/wp/dangerous-terms-users-guide-eulas

62. U.S. FDA. FDA In Brief: FDA Takes New Steps to Advance Risk-Based Regulation of Digital Health Tools. 2018, December 13. Accessed January 2020. https://www.fda.gov/news-events/fda-brief/fda-brief-fda-takes-new-steps-advance-risk-based-regulation-digital-health-tools?rel=0

63. Szabo L. Artificial Intelligence is Rushing into Patient Care and Could Raise Risks. *Scientific American*. 2019, December 24.

64. Thompson SA, and C Warzel. Twelve Million Phones, One Dataset, Zero Privacy. *New York Times*. 2019, December 19.

PART 3
FRAMEWORKS FOR DIGITAL RISK AND THREAT MITIGATION

11
Modeling Cyber Threats as Medical Adverse Events

The magnitude and impact of cyber threats to digital health as described in the 10 Toxicities necessitates designing in mitigations and ongoing surveillance once these technologies are put into practice. Risk management approaches for the 10 Toxicities, and cyber and privacy threats more generally, must account for changes in all aspects of risk including new threats and vulnerabilities, changes to the magnitude in the impact of weaknesses, or new uses for the information technology (IT) system or device.

Failure of imagination, unknown unknowns, and black swans

The science fiction writer and futurist Arthur C. Clarke wrote that "to predict the future we need logic, but we also need faith and imagination which can sometimes defy logic itself."[1] Clarke went on to describe two types of failure of imagination: failure of nerve and failure to admit the possibility of the existence of vital facts. A failure of nerve is a lack of courage to follow "all technical extrapolations to their logical conclusion." Denying the existence of facts that may be revealed, "as the result of new scientific breakthroughs," is a failure in which technological advances are not considered in the development of new knowledge. New technologies must be viewed through this lens in order to reveal the resulting opportunities and threats they pose.

The 21st United States Secretary of Defense, Donald Rumsfeld, famously articulated this concern during a press conference in the wake of the tragic 9/11 attacks, "... as we know, there are known knowns; there are things we know we know. We also know there are known unknowns; that is to say we know there are some things we do not know. But there are also unknown unknowns—the ones we don't know we don't know. And if one looks throughout the history of our country and other free countries, it is the latter category that tend to be the difficult ones."[2]

Digital Health. Eric D. Perakslis and Martin Stanley, Oxford University Press (2021). © Oxford University Press.
DOI: 10.1093/oso/9780197503133.003.0011

Following the Financial Crisis in 2008, Nassim Taleb popularized the phrase "Black Swan" in reference to unforeseen (no/low probability events) having such disproportionately large impact that they must be mitigated against and vigilantly monitored.[3] Whether we call this failure of imagination, unknown unknowns, or black swans, the potential human impact of widespread adverse events or the disruption of care is an intolerable risk that must be accounted for across all threat spaces (cyber, physical, safety, supply chain, etc.) all the while as we adapt and adopt technology breakthroughs. We must consider that the risk landscape can change in unforeseen ways and that threats can develop quicker than we can apply protections. Unknown unknowns could be unforeseen uses of health IT, new vulnerabilities, and changes in the environment in which health IT operates (including the introduction of disruptive technologies).

Impacts from cyber threats must be factored into medical adverse event risk management. Existing cyber risk management approaches such as the Center for Internet Security Top-20 Controls and Resources, NIST Risk Management Framework, and the NIST Cybersecurity Framework provide useful strategies for managing known cyber risks and are a great starting point for supplementing medical benefit-risk determination. These approaches promote building in cybersecurity up front during the design process and adding security controls during the system lifecycle in order to defend against known cybersecurity risks. Few in health care, however, even know of their existence. Managing the trade-offs between the categories of risks that can lead to medical adverse events, now more than ever, requires expertise beyond the medical domain. In my experience, many of the healthcare institutions that are ahead in cybersecurity are so because they borrowed methodologies, or, even better, hired cybersecurity leaders and professionals from other industries.

Regardless, diligence is essential when it comes to cyber risks, particularly as it relates to the magnitude of the damage that could be done as a result of failures to adequately protect systems and data. Measures should be applied in a risk-based manner, meaning they should be considered where the risk of the exploit of a weakness exceeds an organizations risk tolerance. Methods that complement cybersecurity risk management by providing visibility into unknown unknowns include: bug bounty programs, subscription to threat information services, red-teaming, and the MITRE ATT&CK framework. Diligently managing known risks by building in security and monitoring for new threats in this manner will increase the assurance that medical adverse events due to cyber threats are minimized.

Adverse events are impacts in the cyber risk equation

As discussed earlier in the 10 Toxicities of Digital Health, cyber risk management is a critical factor in managing adverse events related to digital health. Cybersecurity risks are commonly described in the following manner:

Risk = Threat × Vulnerability × Impact × Likelihood

Minimizing or eliminating the four factors on the right side of the Risk Management Equation either reduces or eliminates the risk altogether. Each of the 10 Toxicities is itself either a risk, a known vulnerability, or a threat to at least one aspect of the confidentiality, availability, and integrity triad described later; viewing the 10 Toxicities in this manner illuminates measures that may be used to mitigate or eliminate cyber risks. These measures may involve the application of specific classes of cyber protections defined by NIST as technical, management, and operational controls.

In the case of digital health, the IT systems and medical devices used to deliver care are of greatest concern. The impact of a medical adverse event is a common denominator for any risk to a particular health IT system or medical device. The impact has a direct correlation to the magnitude of any particular risk. Threats may come from adversarial or nonadversarial actors who actively or inadvertently exploit a vulnerability that results in an event of some consequence. Vulnerabilities are deficiencies in health IT and medical devices, processes or procedures for their use, or security controls or designs that could be acted on by a threat actor. The chance that threat or vulnerability could be carried out is represented as the likelihood factor in the Cyber Risk Equation. The chapter began with a discussion of unknown unknowns and failure of imagination and their relationship to significant impacts. In many cases low-likelihood scenarios are written off by risk managers or designers in favor of increased functionality, lower cost, speed to market, etc.

All risks are not equal and factors such as consequence and likelihood are used to ensure that the most important risks are differentiated from the trivial. Two major axioms of risk management are that no risk is accepted unnecessarily and that all risk is accepted at the appropriate level of the organization.[4] First, it is not just the risks we know about. We must protect against known risks, but we also must have a strategy to address high-impact, low-probability events, as well as unknown unknowns. Effective management of cybersecurity risks requires more than just skilled cybersecurity professionals. Medical domain subject matter expertise is necessary to continuously monitor for potential risks and to ensure that the security controls, mitigations, and acceptance of risk is done appropriately, in balance with the need to effectively utilize health IT, and to accept the consequences of a compromise. Ensuring that the developers of systems and devices have strong collaboration with security teams during the system development and testing phases is a critical factor to building in and maintaining security. We will detail further the importance of maintaining this collaboration throughout the entire system lifecycle.

Breakdowns in the lifecycle approach to cybersecurity risk management occur when the context and purpose of the system/device is lost. This can happen in many ways. For example, an organization or a regulatory body can apply a one-size-fits-all approach where consequence and likelihood are de-emphasized. Or a *risk-adverse* approach can prevail where checklists of security controls are applied in a manner that limits the functionality of the system, delays its benefit, greatly increases the cost, or creates incentives for designers/users to defeat or disable protections.

To balance the security and functionality of a system NIST provides an elegant way for visualizing impacts of cybersecurity compromises. The Confidentiality, Integrity, and Availability (CIA) Triad represents three high-level cybersecurity *objectives* that broadly address the cybersecurity concerns of system and device stakeholders. These cybersecurity objectives can be subsequently used to categorize the types and magnitude of cybersecurity risks to systems and data. Once the impact level of a health IT system is determined against each of the high-level objectives, the highest impact rating of the three objectives (also known as the "High Water Mark") is used to determine the overall security categorization of the system.

Measuring organizational risk tolerance for a particular IT system or device may be accomplished by applying the Federal Information Processing Standards Publication 199 (FIPS PUB 199), which categorizes the potential impacts related to the CIA Triad into High, Moderate, and Low concerns. For organizations that require additional granularity NIST recently released guidance that further recommends subimpact levels (High, Moderate and Low) at each of the higher-level impact categories.[5] This subcategorization is intended to be used by larger organizations that are looking to prioritize cybersecurity protections across an extensive portfolio of systems.

Threats to health IT and medical devices are aligned with the NIST definitions of the CIA Triad in highly specific ways. First, confidentiality— *preserving authorized restrictions on information access and disclosure, including means for protecting personal privacy and proprietary information are needed*. With respect to health IT and medical devices, confidentiality typically refers to the guarding of protected health information (PHI) as defined under the HIPAA Privacy and Security Rules. The threats to confidentiality are well represented in the 10 Toxicities, particularly as they relate to privacy, physical security, cybercrime, and medical charlatanism. Protecting proprietary information not only preserves commercial advantages but also ensures that proprietary information isn't stolen, copied, and reused in substandard patient care resulting in adverse events, misuse, and reputational risk for the owner of the intellectual property.

Concurrently, availability—the property of being accessible and useable on demand by an authorized entity, is also essential. For health IT and medical devices, availability means that the resource is available and functional to providers and patients. The 10 Toxicities consider concerns which result in systems and devices being unavailable (i.e., care disruption attacks as a result of cybercrime and financial toxicity), or in some cases too available (cyberchondria, overdiagnosis, overtreatment, and medical device deregulation). Availability is often impacted by the application of security protections and can pit users against the security teams. For health IT the rapid pace of technical advancement can result in clinicians and patients lacking sufficient knowledge and training on a system, bringing about medical and/or user error. Usability of a device and preserving functionality must be balanced with protections for confidentiality and integrity.

Integrity refers to guarding against improper information modification or destruction, and includes ensuring information nonrepudiation and authenticity. Integrity is often misunderstood and an afterthought when considering cybersecurity risks. It is possible that this is due to the lack of instances of integrity attacks or the focus on data breaches. Loss of integrity of health data should be considered to be a grave risk to the efficacy and safety of health IT. Within the 10 Toxicities, medical misinformation, physical security, and medical charlatanism represent threats to the integrity of health IT. Medicine is foundationally science based, and if the data or measurements relied upon to make science-based decisions can't be trusted, the efficacy and safety of entire classes of treatment may come into question.

Security categorization and controls

Within the 10 Toxicities the interrelationships of the three categories of threats are complex. Fortunately, there is an approach to determine how to proceed with the application of cyber protections. The security categorization of a system drives the application of security controls. Cybersecurity protections are organized into various baselines according to the overall security categorization of the system (as determined by the "High Water Mark") in NIST SP800-53r5 Security and Privacy Controls for Federal Information Systems and Organization.[6] Additional catalogs of security controls and capabilities are the Center for Internet Security Top-20 Controls and Resources and the NIST Cybersecurity Framework. Within each of these approaches, the initial work to categorize the impact of system compromise drives the selection of security controls and capabilities. Security controls can be technical, management, or operational and these categories parallel the technology, processes, and oversight that are applied in order to achieve safety and efficacy in medicine.

Technical controls are defined as security controls (i.e., safeguards or countermeasures) for an information system that are primarily implemented and executed through mechanisms contained in the hardware, software, or firmware components of the information system.[7] Encryption of data, multifactor authentication, firewalls, and antivirus measures are examples of technical controls.

Management controls are security controls (i.e., safeguards or countermeasures) for an information system that focus on the management of risk and information system security.[8] Risk-review meetings, authorization to operate systems, and leadership review of security metrics in a time or event-based manner are examples of management controls.

Operational controls are security controls (i.e., safeguards or countermeasures) for an information system that are primarily implemented and executed by people (as opposed to systems).[9] Processes and procedures for the use of health IT systems and devices are examples of operational controls.

How do we determine what is a weakness? The primary components of risk with which we are concerned are the identification and management of threats and vulnerabilities related to health IT. Recall the Cybersecurity Risk Management Equation:

Risk = Threat × Vulnerability × Impact × Likelihood

There are many lists of threats and vulnerabilities and threat information resources. A list of known cyber threats to health IT and medical devices is presented below, along with common vulnerabilities. We also present key concepts to consider when designing in security protections and engaging in the ongoing management of cyber risk. Cyber threats are not static and frequently increase over time, both in magnitude of impact and number of potential actors who can exploit a weakness.

Although managing known cyber threats can increase the difficulty of conducting an attack, it does not account for the failures of imagination or the unknown unknowns. The risk of waiting for a threat to be known and remediated creates a continual risk of cyber-based adverse events impacting populations. This is the environment in which health IT now operates. An approach to continuously monitoring the environment(s) in which health IT operates for significant changes based on criticality or the potential impact of adverse events is necessary. The continuous review should include the current and new use(s) of the device, interactions with new technology in the environment that the device operates, and increase/decrease in the reliance of clinicians and patients on the device. For example, an upgrade to an insulin pump may now allow the device to connect to a patient's smartphone, creating an opportunity for an adversary to attack the insulin pump if the smartphone is compromised. The potential for an unknown unknown to disrupt care, cause a medical/user error, or otherwise negatively impact populations is a continual risk that must be accepted.

Risk-based (impact) or threat-based (threat)?

When selecting approaches to apply cybersecurity to health IT, it is important to understand the intended use of these approaches and how the differing regimes can be used in a complementary manner. First and foremost, cybersecurity must be accounted for early in the system-design process and built into health IT. Beyond engineering cybersecurity into health IT, cybersecurity must be an ongoing concern throughout the health IT lifecycle. This ongoing approach must account for the changes to all the factors that constitute the cybersecurity risk equation. Over time, new weaknesses can emerge, likelihoods of exploits can change, and the impact of compromises can increase or decrease. No risk management is perfect, however; organizations must seek to continuously improve their capabilities to identify, mitigate, and accept risks in accordance with the threat they pose balanced by an organization's risk tolerance.

NIST Risk Management Framework (RMF)

The NIST SP800 Series offers a comprehensive approach to Cybersecurity Risk Management. The SP800 Series was originally intended for application in federal IT systems but can be applied universally. Major volumes include The Risk Management Framework (NIST SP800-37r2), an integrated catalog of security and privacy controls (NIST SP800-53r5), and a comprehensive approach for continuous monitoring of the effectiveness of security controls (NIST SP800-137).

Intended to address the common needs of most organizations, the NIST Cybersecurity Framework is a practical and flexible approach to matching security activities and protections to meet particular security *outcomes*. The Framework is organized into five cybersecurity outcomes (Identify, Detect, Protect, Respond, and Recover) and further categorized and subcategorized into various activities and technical approaches intended to achieve these outcomes. The Framework protections are organized into Tiers based on the magnitude of the security concerns associated with the five cybersecurity outcomes. Lastly, the Framework provides specific references for best practice implementations of the security controls that are specified. Building from readily accessible standards, guidelines, and practices, the Framework provides a common taxonomy and mechanism for organizations to: (1) Describe their current cybersecurity posture; (2) Describe their target state for cybersecurity; (3) Identify and prioritize opportunities for improvement within the context of a continuous and repeatable process; (4) Assess progress toward the target state; and (5) Communicate among internal and external stakeholders about cybersecurity risk.

The Risk Management Framework (RMF) outlines a sequence of steps that should be repeated throughout the health IT system lifecycle:

(1) Categorize—Determine the impact of the health IT system and data used by the system

(2) Select—Choose security controls commensurate with the risk of operating a health IT system or device at the relevant impact level

(3) Implement—Implement security controls as part of the design or operation of the health IT system

(4) Assess—Determine how well the security controls meet the protection objectives of the relevant impact level

(5) Authorize—Complete an organizational process to accept the residual risk (risk not mitigated by security controls) and approve the health IT system for operation

(6) Monitor—Periodically review health IT system security controls for efficacy in a dependable, repeatable, and trustworthy process.[10]

These steps should be repeated periodically throughout the lifecycle of the health IT system. The process for determining when to repeat these steps should be risk-based (depending on the impact of the health IT system or device). This risk-based approach can be time-driven or event-based.

An important addition to the latest revision of NIST SP800-37r2 is the introduction of a foundational step called Prepare. The Prepare step is a process that can occur at any time during the system lifecycle to prepare the organization to effectively manage cybersecurity risk. Best completed prior to beginning to manage risk, NIST has recognized that organizations require an approach to build in risk management where it may be lacking in the organization at any time during the system lifecycle.

Traditional cybersecurity risk management approaches have been augmented in recent years by threat-based frameworks that leverage emerging knowledge from threat actor tactics, techniques, and procedures (TTPs) to improve cyber techniques. The value of using a threat-based approach is twofold: (1) Validation that security controls designed into a system protect against new threats; and (2) Ensuring that new weaknesses are identified and addressed throughout the system lifecycle.

After a system is designed to be secure, against known threats at a particular impact level, emerging threats can't wait to be addressed until the next design cycle. Threat-based frameworks are a key component of continuous risk management and are used to identify what additional controls (or modifications to existing controls) should be applied to mitigate specifically against a particular threat. This approach has the added benefit of providing a methodical way to determine the relationship of a particular threat to the security posture of the system or device. The determination to leverage a threat-based framework can be part of the health IT system design approach or be event-based. Aligning threats to health IT and medical devices in the context of the CIA triad more readily enables the application of cybersecurity risk management best practices. The remainder of this chapter categorizes threats to health IT systems and devices used to manage and deliver patient care. Cyber threats to health IT are at the core of the 10 Toxicities. Within this chapter we categorize these threats in several basic categories to make them easier to understand and manage.

Privacy and identity theft

Protected health information (PHI) is desirable to cyber criminals because it can be used to steal identities. Protecting PHI is directly analogous to cybersecurity discipline of protecting the confidentiality of data. Stealing identities and using those identities to conduct fraud is the leading threat to health information. In 2019, 14.4 million people were victims of identity theft.[11] As Healthcare Delivery Organizations (HDO) and Medical Device Manufacturers (MDM) successfully deploy IT platforms and devices that gather and process PHI they must be wary of the threats and potential impacts of this criminal activity. Theft of multiple identities and related Personally Identifiable Information (PII) and PHI allows cyber criminals to access bank accounts, open credit card accounts, and even file false tax returns in pursuit of financial gain. It can take victims significant time and effort to recover from identity theft.

The financial and reputational impact to a company that suffers a loss of PII or PHI can be enormous. According to the Ponemon Institute the average cost of a healthcare associated data breach was $6.45 million.[12] Quantifying reputational damage in monetary terms is not a simple task, but certainly public perception can be negatively impacted for significant periods of time when brands are associated with major breaches. Criminal enterprises often hide behind international boundaries where law enforcement is further challenged to prosecute identity thieves. Jurisdiction is the number one barrier to prosecuting cybercrime.[13] Despite international agreements among law enforcement agencies, the challenges of attribution (identifying the threat actor), gathering court admissible evidence, and differing statutes related to cybercrime are formidable barriers to bringing identity thieves to justice. As a result of these factors identity theft is rampant. Look no further than the U.S. Department of Health and Human Services Office of Civil Rights HIPPA "Wall of Shame," which rank orders the largest HIPPA violations by date, number of affected individuals, and type of breach.[14] Beyond the statutory obligation for HIPAA-covered entities to protect the confidentiality of PHI, the loss of PHI also can result in the loss of an individual's privacy. The disclosure of patients' health information could result in stigma, embarrassment, and discrimination[15] and further expose them to medical charlatanism as described in the 10 Toxicities.

Emerging threats to privacy and identity theft specific to PII and PHI include the increasing number of non-HIPAA-covered entities that are collecting, storing, and using this information for health and wellness services. This includes fitness apps, wearables such as the Apple Watch and Fitbit, and more. The user of these devices may infer protections, rights, and recourse due to the similarity of use or the similarity of information that is being gathered on these platforms to information conveyed in the delivery of care by HIPAA-covered clinicians and health insurance companies.

Care disruption

When applying the CIA triad to health IT a primary objective is determining how important *availability* (being available to be used) is to the health IT system. This determination may be very obvious in some regards, and in others require extensive knowledge of the application of the system or the environment that the device operates in. Care disruption has been and should remain a major concern for medical providers given the numerous ransomware attacks that have plagued large and small clinical sites. The prevalence of these *availability* attacks necessitates consideration of ransomware threats as having a high *likelihood* of being realized. Care disruption could also occur with an *integrity*-based attack. In such a case, care is disrupted because the health IT system can't be counted on to perform accurately or reliably. To date, attacks on the *integrity* of health IT systems have not been prevalent, but just because the *likelihood* of an *integrity* attack is low, the magnitude of the impact that could result may make this an unacceptable risk to simply accept as part of the regular course of business.

The proliferation of digital health is increasing the number of ways that hackers can disrupt care, as well as reducing visibility into the care disruption threat space through increased complexity. The growing reliance on technology in healthcare magnifies the ways in which care could be impeded or disrupted. Furthermore, the interconnected nature of health IT and medical devices coupled with dependencies on common networks, systems, and resources creates an intricate web of virtual connections and shared data just within a small office. Cybersecurity professionals refer to the systems and data exposed to malicious actors as an "attack surface." As a result of this, the rise of technology-enabled medical facilities and devices represents an ever growing, and increasingly complex attack surface for the medical profession to defend.

Care disruptions can comprise: the loss of a single medical device or entire families of devices; the loss of an entire manufacturer due to reliance on core technology such as operating systems; impeded access to systems, records, communication, and staffing coordination; and lack of confidence in proven treatments and/or medical authorities. Cyber risk management must be an integral part of the overall risk management approach to care delivery. Care delivery risk management itself, must be holistic, ensuring protections for the categories of risk (compliance, supply chain, utilities, cybersecurity, etc.) are not applied in an overlapping or conflicting manner.

Healthcare systems and medical devices are targeted due to the value of the data and the potential for care disruption to human patients. These impacts can be quantified through processes such as *categorization* of the health IT System, wherein the use of the health IT system and the value of the data that the system contains drives the protection goals.

The universe and complexity of cyberthreats continues to outpace the efforts of cyberdefenders. The daunting nature of the threat-scape results in most compromises continuing undiscovered for an average of 206 days.[16] During this time period adversaries conduct reconnaissance, ex-filtrate data, and interrupt mission-critical capabilities unabated. More often than not, compromises are not identified by enterprise cybersecurity teams but by third parties who have discovered the malicious activity through other means.

Health IT is subject to the full cyberthreat landscape present in today's interconnected environment. Leading the list of *Known Knowns* and *Known Unknowns* are high-profile ransomware attacks on hospitals and large-scale PHI breaches at health care and insurance providers as reported at the Department of Health and Human Services Office of Civil Rights. We refer to these threats and vulnerabilities as *known knowns* and *known unknowns* because in many cases we know the weakness, the way it may become compromised, and the intent of the adversary. We also use *known unknowns* as these are known weaknesses that ultimately may be used in a way that cannot be predicted.

Brief overview of specific threats

Ransomware targets the availability of critical systems. Ransomware threats are carried out by malicious actors who infiltrate health IT systems and encrypt critical systems and data such that they cannot be accessed without paying the adversary a "ransom" to get the key or passcode to decrypt the data. Often, the ransomware will infiltrate backups and offline backups further limiting the options to restore systems. In many cases it becomes a cost/benefit analysis on whether to pay the ransom. To date, ransomware attacks have been primarily driven by financial gain.

DoS/DDoS attacks also are intended to impact the availability of an Internet-connected resource. These attacks threaten the ability of legitimate users to access health IT systems due to the actions of a malicious cyber threat actor.[17] These actions typically involve the transmission of large amounts of Internet traffic that overwhelms the resources associated with the target system or network.

Advanced Persistent Threats (APTs) target confidentiality, integrity, and availability. The term APT refers to the placement of malware by an adversary on health IT systems within a provider's network in order to conduct reconnaissance on the network, access other systems within the health IT provider or partner network, force systems in the network to malfunction in an intended or unintended manner, steal data, or pursue other nefarious intents. The tactics of an APT involve the infiltration of a health IT provider network and may remain dormant or simply conduct reconnaissance to identify additional targets or opportunities to compromise resources within the network. The risk to the health IT network in many cases is not known until the APT pursues its ultimate objective.

Malware infections target confidentiality, integrity, and availability. Malware infections refer to a broad threat vector related to the placement of unauthorized software on a health IT system. Malware can be delivered through malicious e-mail attachments, infected thumb drives, compromised web sites, file-sharing services, and virtually any resource that is trusted by the health IT System to share files and data. The impact of malware infections can include ransomware attacks, theft of PHI, use of the health IT system for other nefarious purposes including an APT, and use of the health IT system as part of a botnet which conducts DoS or DDoS attacks on other systems. The minimum acceptable protection is to ensure health IT systems are protected with antivirus software and that the antivirus signatures are kept up-to-date.

Lost or stolen devices typically result in targeting of confidentiality and availability. Failure to account for the possibility of the loss or theft of health IT systems certainly affects the availability of the resource for use by the system owner and authorized users and potentially can result in the loss of the information on the health IT system, which can minimally include PHI and proprietary information.

Known vulnerabilities are extensively accounted for elsewhere in locations such as the National Vulnerability Database (NVD), which is maintained by NIST. Security control catalogs included in the NIST Cybersecurity Framework, NIST SP800-53r5, Center for Internet Security (CIS) Top 20, and others, present a multitude of security controls and best approaches for applying them to protect against known vulnerabilities. Groups of security controls deployed to address a particular vulnerability or weakness are referred to as *capabilities*. Cybersecurity capabilities also build and rely on one another to achieve and enhance their respective protection objectives. What follows are descriptions of health IT vulnerabilities and the security capabilities that can remediate them. Common weaknesses that can be mitigated against by application of commonly available cybersecurity capabilities include:

Unauthorized devices and software

A fundamental tenet of cybersecurity is that you can't secure what you don't know you have. The best-practice approach recommended for mitigating this vulnerability is leveraging hardware and software asset management capabilities that mitigate the potential of having unknown devices on the network and unauthorized software operating on those devices. Furthermore, hardware asset management capabilities can ensure that lost or stolen devices are immediately identified in order to take actions to mitigate the impact of this loss.

Lack of configuration management

Lack of control of the configuration of hardware and software in a medical IT system can result in the medical IT system being used in ways that are unforeseen; or, the system can become a ripe target for an APT to use as a launching point for further attacks within the health IT network. These vulnerabilities are mitigated against by maintaining configuration control over all hardware and software on the network. This may include establishing gold images (common versions of operating systems and applications) that cannot be modified by the user, restricting administrator access, and centralized monitoring of the configuration settings of health IT devices and alerting incident response staff of any changes to these settings.

Lack of vulnerability management

Most compromises of IT systems are a result of a known unpatched vulnerability. Not patching a known vulnerability is a cardinal sin of cybersecurity risk management. In 2019, the Ponemon Institute reported that 60% of breach respondents stated that a patch was available for a known vulnerability but not applied.[18] There is no substitute for, and no excuse for not, monitoring the availability of patches for health IT systems and applying them in a timely fashion. Vulnerability management leverages an accurate inventory of systems and software on the network so that vulnerabilities can be identified when they are reported; it also leverages vulnerability scanning capabilities to detect when vulnerabilities have remained undetected, and strong change-control processes to ensure that patches for vulnerabilities are deployed in a timely and risk-based manner.

Access control/identity management

Ensuring that health IT devices and data are only accessible to authorized users is a critical capability to guarantee all aspects of the CIA Triad. Like most cybersecurity capabilities, access control and identity management are reliant on hardware/software asset inventories to ensure that access is restricted on all health IT devices and systems. Access control is most commonly maintained as a username/password combination. Protecting health IT systems with us-ername/password combinations only is *highly insecure* and very risky. The increase in interconnected health IT systems magnifies this risk.

Identity management goes hand in hand with access control and is necessary to ensure that health IT Systems are accessed only by authorized users. The most secure access control system can be defeated by impersonating the identity of an authorized user. Extensive literature is available regarding the application of user identification and access control best practices. As with other security controls, access control capabilities should be applied in a risk-based manner with additional factors such as one-time tokens and biometrics utilized to protect high-impact data and systems. This control poses a particularly challenging situation for health care. Many clinical systems require immediate or even emergency access. Clinicians often will not have time to use multifactor authentication or something similar, so a balance must be struck. Unfortunately, when the balance leans toward convenience, this places systems at higher risk than is technically necessary.

Zero trust

Legacy health IT networks have been traditionally protected by strong perimeter security controls such as firewalls, virtual private networks, and intrusion detection/prevention systems. As the awareness of the prevalence of APTs has risen, strategies to prevent the propagation of an APT once it has gained a foothold now must be adopted. This capability is commonly referred to as "zero trust." Zero trust means that users, devices, systems, and software are not automatically trusted just because they are connected to a protected network or owned by the same enterprise. If you are protecting digital health systems and data on your network, or using a hybrid of enterprise and cloud-based services, it is recommended that security-design professionals be involved in the application of zero trust techniques to protect against all manner of threats, and to increase the resilience of systems that are compromised.

Data protection

Health IT systems are targeted by malicious actors primarily for their PII records and in the case of an APT, proprietary intellectual property. The best protection for the loss of data and intellectual property is to encrypt this information at all times. This means that at baseline, data should be encrypted in the databases where it is stored, on the systems and devices where it is gathered and used, and on the networks where it is transmitted. Additionally, the application of a Data Loss Prevention (DLP) solution can identify incidents where data has potentially leaked out of the organizational boundaries. When the impact of a data loss event is high, system engineers with extensive experience designing highly secure systems should be involved from the beginning of the design process to ensure that decrypted data for authorized use can't be accessed by an adversary or unauthorized user.

Incident response

Based on all available data, cybersecurity incidents and breaches should be expected and the capabilities to deal with the most common threats and vulnerabilities should be built in and managed by following one of the widely available cybersecurity risk management approaches. In addition to building secure systems and maintaining vigilance to identify new threats and patch known vulnerabilities, health IT systems should be covered by an incident response plan. The incident response plan should minimally include preparing the organization to handle incidents, detecting and analyzing security data and incidents, mitigating incidents when they occur, and determining appropriate follow-up actions such as application of additional security controls or mitigations to protect against future recurrences.[19]

In a case study, vulnerabilities specific to wireless infusion pumps, which generalize well to all medical devices, were gathered by researchers at the

NIST Cybersecurity Center of Excellence and documented in NIST Special Publication 1800-8 Securing Wireless Infusion Pumps in Healthcare Delivery Organizations.[20]

Long useful life: Infusion pumps are designed to perform clinical functions for several years, and they tend to have long-term refresh rates. One vulnerability associated with infrequent refresh is that each device's technological attributes may become obsolete or insufficient to support patching or updating, or cybersecurity controls that may become available in the future.

Information/data vulnerabilities:

Lack of encryption on private/sensitive data at rest: Pump devices may have local persistent storage, but they may not have a means to encrypt data stored on the device. Locally stored data may include sensitive configuration information, or patient information, including possible PHI.

Lack of encryption on transmitted data: Sensitive data should be safeguarded in transit as well as at rest. Where capabilities exist, pumps and server components should employ encryption on the network or when transmitting sensitive information. An inability to safeguard data in transit, by using appropriate encryption capabilities, may expose sensitive information or allow malicious actors to determine how to connect to a pump or server to perform unauthorized activities.

Insufficient data backup: Providing backup and recovery capability is a common cybersecurity control to ensure that healthcare delivery organizations (HDOs) can restore services in a timely fashion after an adverse event. Hospitals should perform appropriate pump system backup and restore functions.

Lack of capability to de-identify private/sensitive data: As a secondary cybersecurity control to data encryption, hospitals may wish to consider the ability to de-identify or obfuscate sensitive information or PHI.

Lack of data validation: Data used and captured by infusion pumps and associated server components may require data integrity assurance to support proper functioning and patient safety. Mechanisms should be used to provide assurance that data cannot be altered inappropriately.

Device/endpoint (infusion pump) vulnerabilities:

Debug-enabled interfaces: Interfaces required to support or troubleshoot infusion pump functions should be identified, with procedures noted to indicate when interfaces are available, and how interfaces may be disabled when not required for troubleshooting or system updates/fixes.

Use of removable media: Infusion pumps that include external or removable storage should be identified. Cybersecurity precautions are necessary because the use of removable media may lead to inappropriate information disclosure and may provide a viable avenue for malicious software to migrate to the pump or server components.

Lack of physical tamper detection and response: Infusion pumps may involve physical interaction, including access to interfaces used for debugging. HDOs should enable mechanisms to prevent physical tampering with infusion pump devices, including alerting appropriate personnel whenever a pump or its server components are manipulated or altered.

Misconfiguration: Mechanisms should be used to ensure that pump configurations are well-managed and may not be configured to produce adverse conditions.

Poorly protected and patched devices: Like the misconfiguration vulnerability, HDOs should implement processes to protect/patch/update pumps and server components. This may involve including controls on the device, or provisions that allow for external controls that would prevent exposure to flaws or weaknesses.

User or administrator accounts vulnerabilities:

Hard-coded or factory-default passcodes: Processes or mechanisms should be added to prevent the use of so-called hard-coded or factory-default passcodes. This would overcome a common information-technology (IT) systems deficiency in the use of authentication mechanisms for privileged access to devices, in terms of using weak passwords or passcodes protection. Weak authentication mechanisms that are well-known or published degrade the effectiveness of authentication control measures. HDOs should implement a means to update and manage passwords.

Lack of role-based access and/or use of principles of least privilege: When access management roles and principles of least privilege are poorly designed, they may allow the use of a generic identity (e.g., a so-called admin account) that enables a greater access capability than necessary. HDOs should implement processes to limit access to privileged accounts, infusion pumps, and server components, and should use accounts or identities that tie to specific functions, rather than providing/enabling the use of super user, root, or admin privileges.

Dormant accounts: Accounts or identities that are not used may be described as dormant. Dormant account information should be disabled or removed from pumps and server components.

Weak remote access controls: When remote access to a pump and/or server components is required, access controls should be appropriately enforced to safeguard each network session and to ensure appropriate authentication and authorization.

Secure design

Designing-in cybersecurity protections against these common threats and vulnerabilities often has been an afterthought by system engineers, well beyond just the realm of health IT. Comprehensive approaches to system security engineering are now becoming available. In particular, NIST has released the first two volumes of NIST SP800-160 Systems Security Engineering. NIST SP800-160v1 adapts 30 ISO/IEC engineering processes to systems security engineering in a flexible approach that can be adopted across a systems lifecycle. These processes focus on the steps an organization should take at critical phases of the system lifecycle and is not prescriptive with respect to the security controls that should be applied.

DevSecOps refers to a systematic approach that embeds security testing and design into the development process. Instilling a DevSecOps approach has a proven track record of reducing the cost of a data breach by $10.55 per compromised record. Furthermore, a DevSecOps approach, on average, can dramatically reduce the time a development team takes to fix a vulnerability found in software (from 174 days to just 92 days).[21]

In addition, bug bounty programs, as the name suggests, involves offering payment to cybersecurity researchers who identify and report vulnerabilities in health IT systems. This has become a best practice and should be applied to health IT systems that are widely deployed and/or where the impact associated with compromise are high. Other facets of security-by-design are "red teaming" and penetration testing. In order to increase the safety of medical devices, at the 2019 cybersecurity conference Def Con, 10 of the top medical device companies permitted the top ethical hackers to attempt to compromise medical devices for the purpose of identifying weaknesses. These weaknesses could then be mitigated by the manufacturers prior to potentially becoming the cause of an adverse event.[22] This approach of systematically testing the security of devices by leveraging "red teams" to conduct penetration tests of medical devices can reduce the time that an adversary has to leverage a vulnerability for malicious purposes and increase the safety and security of health IT.

References

1. Clark AC. Hazards of Prophecy: The Failure of Imagination. 1962s.l. HMH.
2. wikiquote. Accessed December 2019. https://en.wikiquote.org/wiki/Donald_Rumsfeld.
3. Taleb N. *The Black Swan: The Impact of the Highly Improbable*. s.l. : Random House, 2007.
4. United States Department of the Army. Risk Management—Army Publishing Directorate. armypubs.army.mil. 2014. https://armypubs.army.mil/epubs/DR_pubs/DR_a/pdf/web/atp5_19.pdf.
5. National Institute of Standards and Technology. *NIST SP800-37, Revision 2: Risk Management Framework for Information Systems and Organizations*. Gaithersburg, MD: Author, 2018.
6. *NIST Special Publication 800-53 Revision 4: Security and Privacy Controls for Federal Information Systems*. Gaithersburg, MD: National Institute of Standards and Technology, 2013.
7. National Institute of Standards and Technology. Federal Information Processing Standards Publication 200. nist.gov. 2006, March. https://nvlpubs.nist.gov/nistpubs/FIPS/NIST.FIPS.200.pdf.
8. National Institute of Standards and Technology. Federal Information Processing Standards Publication 200. nist.gov. 2006, March. https://nvlpubs.nist.gov/nistpubs/FIPS/NIST.FIPS.200.pdf.
9. National Institute of Standards and Technology. Federal Information Processing Standards Publication 200. nist.gov. 2006, March. https://nvlpubs.nist.gov/nistpubs/FIPS/NIST.FIPS.200.pdf.
10. National Institute of Standards and Technology. NIST Special Publication 800-37 Revision 2: Risk Management Framework for Information Systems and Organizations. 2018, December. https://nvlpubs.nist.gov/nistpubs/SpecialPublications/NIST.SP.800-37r2.pdf.
11. LaPonsie M. 10 Things to Do After Your Identity Is Stolen. 2019. usnews.com. https://money.usnews.com/money/personal-finance/family-finance/articles/things-to-do-after-your-identity-is-stolen.
12. IBM and The Ponemon Institute. *2019 Cost of a Data Breach Report*. Traverse City: Ponemon Institute, 2019.
13. Grimes, Roger A. Why It's So Hard to Prosecute Cyber Criminals. CSO Online. 2016. https://www.csoonline.com/article/3147398/why-its-so-hard-to-prosecute-cyber-criminals.html.
14. HHS OCR. Breach Portal: Notice to the Secretary of HHS Breach of Unsecured Protected Health Information. U.S. Department of Health and Human Services Office for Civil Rights. 2019. https://ocrportal.hhs.gov/ocr/breach/breach_report.jsf.
15. Nass SJ, Levit LA, Gostin LO (Eds.). Beyond the HIPAA Privacy Rule: Enhancing Privacy, Improving Health Through Research. nih.gov. 2009. https://www.ncbi.nlm.nih.gov/books/NBK9579/.
16. IBM and Ponemon Institute. *2019 Cost of A Data Breach Report*. North Traverse City: Ponemon Institute, 2019.
17. Peters J. What is a DDoS Attack? Identifying Denial-of-Service Attacks. varonis.com., 2019, September 25. https://varonis.com/blog/what-is-a-ddos-attack/.
18. Ponemon Institute and ServiceNow. *Costs and Consequences of Gaps in Vulnerability Response*. Traverse City: Ponemon Institute, 2019.
19. National Institute of Standards and Technology. *NIST Special Publication 800-61: Computer Security Incident Handling Guide*. Gaithersburg, MD: Author, 2012.

20. National Institute of Standards and Technology. *NIST Special Publication 1800-8: Securing Wireless Infusion Pumps in Healthcare Delivery Organizations*. Gaithersburg, MD: Author, 2018.

21. Drinkwater D. What Is DevSecOps? Developing More Secure Applications. CSO Online. 2018. https://www.csoonline.com/article/3245748/what-is-devsecops-developing-more-secure-applications.html.

22. Marks J. The Cybersecurity 202: Hackers Are Going After Medical Devices—And Manufacturers Are Helping Them. washingtonpost.com. 2019, August 8. https://www.washingtonpost.com/news/powerpost/paloma/the-cybersecurity-202/2019/08/08/the-cybersecurity-202-hackers-are-going-after-medical-devices-and-manufacturers-are-helping-them/5d4b556088e0fa4cc4c23465/.

12

Current State of Cyber Regulation

Understanding Privacy versus Security

Although regulations for privacy and security have different origins, it is increasingly being recognized that these disciplines share many complementary facets and should be integrated wherever possible. That said, it is important to understand the objectives of privacy and security to ensure both are being met as required and to best prepare for the technology transformations that are disrupting the existing regulatory regime. The simple fact is that there is no digital safety net today and well-intentioned "fixes" can themselves be vectors for the 10 Toxicities.

Privacy

Privacy is discussed often but our expectations and understanding of privacy often lack commonality and foundation. The Bill of Rights offers no express mention of the right to privacy although elements related to privacy, such as the Fourth Amendment right to be free from unreasonable searches and seizures, are frequently interpreted as protecting privacy.[1] Other aspects of the Bill of Rights can be similarly interpreted but the lack of a specific mention, definition, and protection for privacy makes the constitutional basis for privacy murky. Practically speaking the founding fathers could not have imagined a time when personal information could be available instantly to anyone, anywhere. Furthermore, the idea of privacy with respect to other rights (such as seizure or prosecution) or entities (government and healthcare providers) is more easily understood than is the fundamental nature of privacy. We understand the nature of the impacts of the loss of privacy, but we have trouble placing a specific value on privacy itself.

As technology has transformed society, the trading of private information for convenience and benefit is increasingly prevalent and poorly understood. Modern origins for privacy can be traced back to the Privacy Act of 1974.[2] Broadly speaking, the Privacy Act protects the data that the federal government collects and uses in the course of governing the nation by establishing

Digital Health. Eric D. Perakslis and Martin Stanley, Oxford University Press (2021). © Oxford University Press.
DOI: 10.1093/oso/9780197503133.003.0012

protections against unauthorized disclosures, by provision of a citizen's rights to ensure correct information and to be notified of disclosure. Just as other current laws were also designed to address collection and storage of structured data by government, business, and other organizations, privacy laws were developed as a series of responses to specific concerns, resulting in a checkerboard of federal and state laws, common law jurisprudence, and public and private enforcement that has built up over more than a century.[3]

This approach was similarly applied to health information when the Privacy Rule was established as part of HIPAA. This rule establishes national standards to protect individuals' medical records and other personal health information and applies to health plans, healthcare clearinghouses, and those healthcare providers who conduct certain healthcare transactions electronically. The Rule requires appropriate safeguards to protect the privacy of personal health information and sets limits and conditions on the uses and disclosures that may be made of such information without patient authorization. The Privacy Rule also affords patients rights over their health information, including rights to examine and obtain a copy of their health records, as well as to request corrections.[4]

It is essential to understand, however, that there is no statute or regulation for privacy among individual parties in the U.S. Antidiscrimination and civil liberties statutes instead create a protection mechanism against the impacts of practices that unfairly discriminate against individuals on the basis of certain characteristics (religion, gender, sexual orientation, etc.). Privacy is protected in different contexts in vastly different ways propagating the lack of common understanding, expectations, and value placed on privacy. As a result of technology innovation, we find ourselves in a circumstance in which individuals and groups have, and can access, extensive information about individuals in order to determine what kinds of advertisements they see, what free services they are offered, and to improve the features on the personal devices they purchase. The exchange of private information for these purposes is generally considered beneficial in the sense that individuals have rapid and/or free access to services. In fact, the operators of these services have free rein to leverage this private information in multitudes of ways. This results in businesses being able to set the terms under which they collect and share data.[5] There is a great discrepancy between this model and what is required of healthcare providers under HIPAA. Furthermore, as unregulated collectors of information encroach on borderline HIPAA-covered use cases, they may even achieve commercial advantages in the healthcare provider and/or medical device space despite not being considered a "covered entity." Looking closer at these cases we find that the information gathered by unregulated collectors of information could be more valuable and sensitive than the information that is protected for a covered entity.

Security

Cybersecurity is the practice of protecting computer systems and devices from threats and vulnerabilities regarding their confidentiality, integrity, and availability. Similar to privacy, cybersecurity law and regulation is nascent and typically focused on known knowns; it struggles when presented with unknown unknowns that are obvious in hindsight as technology has evolved. These surprises include the rapid growth of ransomware, deep fakes, and the spread of misinformation on social media platforms. Cybersecurity first became mainstream with the growth of the Internet. One of the first pop culture references to the threat of hackers was in Clifford Stoll's seminal novel, *The Cuckoo's Egg*, in which he described his experience tracking down a hacker who had infiltrated the computer system at the Lawrence Berkeley National Laboratory (LBNL).[6] *The Cuckoo's Egg* describes events that began in 1986 and involved technologists who had deep knowledge of the systems being attacked. Thirty years later, the average technology user may be better informed about cybersecurity risks, but the attackers retain an increasing advantage.

Integrated privacy and security

The weaknesses and inefficiencies in separate protection regimes for both privacy and security having been recognized, a number of integrated approaches are currently being implemented. In the European Union (EU) comprehensive regulation covering data protection and privacy called General Data Protection Regulation (GDPR) is being applied to all entities that collect and utilize EU citizen data. This regulation focuses on the relationship between the individual and the entity that is collecting the data, regardless of purpose. This levels the playing field and reduces the opportunities for nonhealth IT to erode traditional health IT use cases through gaps in the regulatory framework. The United States has yet to adopt or offer a complementary approach to GDPR and is currently using the existing regulatory framework to manage the impacts and implications of entities collecting U.S. citizen data. Prospectively and constructively, the National Institute of Standards and Technology (NIST) has updated its catalog of IT-system security controls (NIST SP 800-53r5) to fully incorporate the controls necessary to protect security and privacy at various impact levels into a common approach. Although this approach applies by statute only to the federal government under FISMA 2014, the NIST SP 800 series is a widely accepted best practice for the protection of IT systems and offers a technical approach to preserving privacy and security in an integrated manner.

Part of the challenge lies in the frequent misunderstanding of privacy as opposed to security. A solid consumer-level literacy example is provided by Norton,

> Privacy and security are related. Privacy relates to any rights you have to control your personal information and how it's used. Think about those privacy policies you're asked to read and agree to when you download new smartphone apps. Security, on the other hand, refers to how your personal information is protected. Your data—different details about you—may live in a lot of places. That can challenge both your privacy and your security. Some people regard privacy and security as pretty much the same thing. That's because the two sometimes overlap in a connected world. But they aren't the same and knowing how they differ may help you to protect yourself in an increasingly connected world.[7]

Compliance versus security and quality versus compliance

Compliance and security are easily conflated and frequently misunderstood. From our earlier publication on this topic in *Science Translational Medicine*,

> First, compliance does not equal security, and the differences and relationships between them are easily misunderstood. Security is the application of protections and management of risk posed by cyber threats. Compliance is typically a top-down mandate based on federal guidelines or law, whereas security is often managed bottom-up and is decentralized in most organizations. Compliance processes typically revolve around documentation, whereas security processes are embedded within the technology life cycle as systems are acquired, used, and discarded.[8]

As a rule of thumb, compliance should be viewed as the application of quality controls, including security controls, as prescribed by statute or regulation, whereas cybersecurity is the management of risks as a result of utilizing technology. Compliance has the advantage of ensuring that the stakeholders of health IT have a common level of assurance related to the protections that should be applied to the health IT systems upon which they rely. Another area to clarify are the challenges of distinguishing quality and compliance. Defining quality is actually quite complex, given that there are simply too many possible ways to accomplish it, depending on what type of quality you are trying to achieve. Approaches include transcendent, product-based, user-based, manufacturing-based, and value-based.[9] Typically, the quality of medical products has been defined at the product and manufacturing level. Product quality often utilizes attributes based on ingredients and inherent attributes, such as durability. Manufacturing-based quality definitions are primarily focused upon engineering and manufacturing practice and what is most well-described and thought of in biomedical product regulation. For example, GXP compliance is rooted in ensuring product quality; however, things don't always work out that way. The problem is that it has become possible to be compliant with regulations on systems that are not high quality. Specifically, many organizations focus on compliance documentation more than actual quality engineering and processes.

Keeping up with digital transformation

We've reiterated throughout this text that the management of security and privacy matters related to digital medicine primarily focuses on safety and efficacy. We also have described a number of related concerns regarding how threats from the technology domain are being inherited by digital health in the form of the 10 Toxicities. Because digital health reflects the sweeping transformation of society, every effort to foster and promote, or to manage the risks brought about by digitization, bears importance in the consideration of digital health. Consider that Amazon could be the new pharmacy, Apple the primary source of health data, Google the new first stop in the healthcare system for patients, and Facebook the new reference for medical facts. What if all these changes occur at the same time? What would that look like? This is all possible. In this world, how will clinicians, patients, and payers fit in? There is much to consider.

Digital transformation is occurring through technology advances in Cloud computing, 5G, the Internet of Things (IoT) devices, artificial intelligence (AI), and quantum computing. With respect to digital health, the infinite possibilities in which they may be applied stand-alone, or in combination, magnifies the complexity of the benefit-risk determination. Furthermore, there are new players (or new to healthcare) who are providing services, regulating these technologies, or using them and their weaknesses, to threaten us. The blending of these trends impacts stakeholders and regulators who often are being faced with transformations that were never considered in rule making and oversight authority. It is increasingly bringing together regulators from different domains who haven't had reason to interact in the past.[10] Such technology transformations can take forms similar to arbitrage in financial markets, in which inefficiencies are advantaged primarily to make profits. Furthermore, new adversaries often are inherited with little awareness of stakeholders. This will grow complexity and opacity as these trends advance, while the underlying technologies, interconnections, and approaches to deliver them surge.

Federal consumer protection regulation

Consumer regulation of products, services, and privacy occurs in the U.S. at the federal level through several authorities:

- The Federal Trade Commission (FTC) protects consumers through its Bureau of Consumer Protection. This bureau focuses primarily on deception, fraud, and unfair practices, all of which propagate the 10 Toxicities. As an example, the FTC initiated actions against online sellers of personal protective equipment during the ongoing 2020 COVID-19 pandemic.[11]
- The Department of Commerce engages in efforts to promote job creation and economic growth. Specific efforts foster commerce, promote technologies, and regulate industries which underlie digital health.[12] These efforts are extensive and relate to the regulation of trade, measurement of economic activity, development of standards, protection of intellectual property, and advising the administration on telecommunications and information policy.
- The Consumer Product Safety Commission (CPSC), "protects the public from unreasonable risks of injury or death associated with the use of the thousands of types of consumer products."[13] The CPSC issued COVID-19 Home Safety Guidance in 2020 to protect consumers from being exposed to or transmitting COVID-19 during the pandemic. Without question, the CPSC will regulate devices that will either be part of the digital health environment by direct connection to digital health devices or involved in the interaction of patients and clinicians with these devices.

- The Department of Transportation is major player in the regulation of technology with a focus on ensuring the safety and utility of the nation's mobility.[14] Autonomous vehicles, unmanned aerial systems, and position, navigation, and timing systems are all examples.
- The Federal Communications Commission (FCC) regulates the nation's communications networks and ensures that the public good is served by government efforts to protect this infrastructure. Actions by the FCC related to next-generation 5G technologies may have an outsized impact on digital health, given that 5G will massively transform how devices communicate through ad hoc networking, on-demand bandwidth, and greater speeds and capacity.[15]
- The Department of Veterans Affairs (VA) is the largest integrated healthcare system in the Unites States.[16] As such, technology advancements at the VA can impact healthcare delivery more broadly, as has been the case with the adoption of electronic health records.
- Department of Homeland Security (DHS) is charged with protecting the nation against all manner of hazards, including cybersecurity threats. The Cybersecurity and Infrastructure Security Agency (CISA) executes the DHS mission to protect against digital and physical threats we face today and to build a more secure and resilient infrastructure for the future.[17]

Executive orders and new laws

The complex landscape of regulation and laws related to health care and associated weaknesses exposed by digital health are described above. In the United States, Congress has the express authority to create new federal laws, as does each state to create new state laws. New laws and the regulation of digital technologies will impact digital health, but may not be driven by digital health concerns, such as the banning of Chinese communications manufacturer Huawei from Universal Service Fund purchase[18] and the Trump Administration Executive Order to address the threat posed by Chinese social media platform TikTok.[19.] It may be tempting to conclude that these occurrences are unrelated to health care, but the close connection between the missions of these regulators and the historical difficulties faced when they must adapt to technology transformation are key challenges that must be managed. Delivery of inaccurate information, lack of understanding of what domain these bodies oversee, and/or subtle differences in messaging alone may be sufficient to further the 10 Toxicities.

References

1. Your Bill of Rights: Your Fourth Amendment Right to Privacy. *Time.* Accessed October 2019. http://content.time.com/time/specials/packages/article/0,28804,2080345_2080344_2080374,00.html

2. United States Department of Justice. Privacy Act of 1974. Accessed October 2019. https://www.justice.gov/opcl/privacy-act-1974

3. Kerry C. Why Protecting Privacy Is a Losing Game Today—And How to Change the Game. 2018, July 12. https://www.brookings.edu/research/why-protecting-privacy-is-a-losing-game-today-and-how-to-change-the-game/.

4. HHS. The HIPAA Privacy Rule. 2015, April 16. Accessed December 2019. https://www.hhs.gov/hipaa/for-professionals/privacy/index.html#:~:targetText=The%20HIPAA%20Privacy%20Rule%20establishes,certain%20health%20care%20transactions%20electronically

5. Kerry C. Why Protecting Privacy Is a Losing Game Today—And How to Change the Game. 2018, July 12. https://www.brookings.edu/research/why-protecting-privacy-is-a-losing-game-today-and-how-to-change-the-game/.

6. Stoll C. *The Cuckoo's Egg: Tracking a Spy Through the Maze of Computer Espionage.* Pocket Books, New York, New York, 2005.

7. Norton by Symantec. Privacy vs. Security: What's the Difference? Norton Security Center. Accessed January 2020. https://us.norton.com/internetsecurity-privacy-privacy-vs-security-whats-the-difference.html

8. Perakslis ED, and M Stanley. A Cybersecurity Primer for Translational Research. *Science Translational Medicine.* 2016. 8(322):322ps2. doi:10.1126/scitranslmed.aaa4493

9. Garvin DA. What Does Product Quality Really Mean? *MIT Sloan Management Review.* 1984, October 15.

10. Pollman E. Tech, Regulatory Arbitrage, and Limits. *European Business Organization Law Review* 2019. 20:567–590. Accessed August 2020. https://link.springer.com/article/10-1007/s40804-019-00155-x

11. Federal Trade Commission. FTC Acts Against Online Sellers Falsely Promised Fast Delivery. Accessed August 2020. https://www.ftc.gov/news-events/press-releases/2020/08/ftc-acts-against-online-sellers-falsely-promised-fast-delivery

12. U.S. Department of Commerce. Learn Grants. Accessed August 2020. https://www.grants.gov/learn-grants/grant-making-agencies/department-of-commerce.html

13. Consumer Product Safety Commission. About CPSC. Accessed August 2020. https://www.cpsc.gov/About-CPSC

14. Department of Transportation. Safety and Health. Accessed August 2020. https://www.transportation.gov/policy/transportation-policy/safety

15. Federal Communications Commission. The FCC's 5G FAST Plan. Accessed August 2020. https://www.fcc.gov/5G

16. Veterans Health Administration. About VHA. Accessed August 2020. https://www.va.gov/health/aboutvha.asp#:~:text=The%20Veterans%20Health%20Administration%20(VHA,Veterans%20enrolled%20in%20the%20VA

17. Cybersecurity and Infrastructure Security Agency. About CISA. Accessed August 2020. https://www.cisa.gov/about-cisa

18. Kelly M. FCC Designates Huawei, ZTE as Risks to National Security. *The Verge*. 2020, June 30. Accessed August 2020. https://www.theverge.com/2020/6/30/21308477/fcc-huawei-zte-ban-universal-service-fund-national-security-threat-risk

19. White House. Executive Order on Addressing the Threat Posed by TikTok. 2020, August 6. Accessed August 2020. https://www.whitehouse.gov/presidential-actions/executive-order-addressing-threat-posed-tiktok/

13

Cybertime

The Key Advantage of the Adversary

Due to the vast number of high-profile cyberattacks, cyberthreats are now deeply present within the psyche of all industries and within our private lives. The response has been explosive, fueling rapid increases in technology spending, calls for increased regulation, for cyber workforce expansion, cyberinsurance, and use of risk management strategies. For any of these to be effective, the math, specifically the impact and realities of time, must be studied very carefully. With hundreds of new attacks launched each minute, traditional risk-management approaches cannot keep up and are proving inadequate. Cyberthreats are vectors having magnitude and direction, and cyberresilience strategies also must be designed as such. By using time as the critical driver, control element, and measure of cybersecurity efficacy, healthcare organizations can prioritize and focus to protect their patients, customers, and themselves.

There is an old expression in agriculture that the best time to plant a tree was 20 years ago. The second-best time is today. This is exactly the situation we have with respect to healthcare cybersecurity. The systems we use today simply were not designed, built, or managed, for the types of advanced persistent threats that exist today. There are many ways that cybersecurity and cyberresilience can be approached and optimized, but the most important factor is time. The majority of systems supporting critical healthcare missions were developed over the course of years or even decades. Major revisions and new features are developed over the course of months and years. Fixes and updates are typically delivered monthly or as emergency releases. System operators extend the time to achieve these system improvements with testing, validation, updates, and patches to ensure functionality and minimum unintended consequences. This extended lifecycle makes it impossible for most organizations to stay up to speed with cyberdefense.

When technology lifecycles, cyberthreat, and cyberdefense are examined from the perspective of time, the facts are striking and can be more easily considered when viewed as three distinct reference frames: technology time,

Digital Health. Eric D. Perakslis and Martin Stanley, Oxford University Press (2021). © Oxford University Press.
DOI: 10.1093/oso/9780197503133.003.0013

cyberthreat time, and regulatory and standards time. Table 13.1 compares the elements of cybertime in 2017, which was chosen as a reference frame due to the occurrence of WannaCry and other high-profile cyber events that year.[1]

Technology time is easily quantified with readily available data. Taking the most common operating systems (OS) as an example, most organizations running Microsoft operating systems are at least one major upgrade behind and are at least five years old. Further, most OS security patch releases are for systems older than seven years. This means that, as systems age, security risk and the corresponding effort required for security patching also increase, adding to cost of ownership, a critical irony given that most system upgrades are delayed due to financial and resource constraints.

The next dimension is cyberthreat time. Here the picture is even more compelling as the denominator shifts from months and years to seconds. With two to three new malware samples being captured and 67 new attacks being launched each second of every day it is very easy for an organization to feel overwhelmed. Resistance to cyberthreats is not steeped in futility, however.

Table 13.1 Cybertime in 2017

Technology Time	*7 years or older*: age of systems for 61% of daily MS security updates
	5 years or older: age of 69.82% of current MS operating instances
	100–120 days: average long time from receipt-to-installation of a security patch
	Daily: an average of 15 security patches are received
	Daily: 44% of security operations managers see at least 5,000 security updates
Cyberthreat Time	*8 months–3 years*: duration of average zero-day attack
	310 days: how long cybercriminals know about a hacker-discovered-vulnerability before the public or vendor
	Weekly: 1–2 zero-day vulnerability are exploited
	2–3 days: a new adobe vulnerability is discovered
	Daily: 200,000 new malware samples are captured
	Daily: 4,000 new ransomware attacks
	Minute: 400 new threats (of all types) are launched
Regulatory & Standards Time	*3–8 years*: average time between federal cyberlaw updates since HIPAA (1996)
	2 years: time between significant updates to NIST cyber/guides standards
	1 year: time from commission-to-repeat of the HHS Healthcare Cyber Task Force

Successful strategies must focus on approaches that stay ahead of the curve but that also can remove time as the denominator of the risk equations. Lastly, with respect to regulatory and standards time, regulations and standards, laws, and policies are developed over far longer time periods, with average historical update time frames at 3.8 and 2 years respectively. Yet, following each high-profile cyberattack, there are renewed calls for more regulation and standards.[2] Although standards and better regulation are essential, they do not occur within time frames that provide defensive utility. First, although never perfect, excellent standards do exist and are being well utilized by the more up-to-date organizations, the strongest examples being the previously discussed National Institute of Standards and Technology (NIST) standards. Second, regulations ultimately serve well only as codification of liability and compliance versus being proactively defensive. Third, as standards and regulations are developed by consensus and subject to public debate, adversaries see these countermeasures coming long before they arrive and can actually use them to design new attack vectors. This leaves mission owners with security solutions that are late to the game and/or ineffective. In contrast, adversaries and cyberactors are acting in hours and minutes against vulnerabilities and weaknesses that are virtually unknown to those who rely on secure and properly functioning IT systems. Adversaries are not constrained by regulation and policy and. are advantaged and emboldened by jurisdictional uncertainties as well as differing laws across national boundaries.

Quantifying risk with time as the denominator

The ancient Chinese general and philosopher Sun Tzu stated, "Strategy without tactics is the slowest route to victory. Tactics without strategy is the noise before defeat." John Boyd, Colonel USAF, developed the decision cycle commonly referred to as the OODA Loop (Observe, Orient, Decide, and Act) to analyze combat air tactics for advantages. Boyd's approach stresses "getting inside" an adversary's decision cycle and tactics (i.e., turning earlier and faster or firing quicker or more accurately).[3] In cybertime this translates to maintaining "time as the denominator" when it comes to interrupting an adversary's decision cycle through defense-in-depth and real-time response to threats and vulnerabilities. Although somewhat simplified, according to Boyd, the side that completes the OODA loop the quickest, wins.

The enterprise approach for Information Security Continuous Monitoring is focused on providing actionable communication of security status.[4] Simply stated, the strategy is based on organizational risk tolerance and is informed by real-time metrics that promote timely responses. Continuous monitoring strategies are based on prioritization of organization assets and functions so that appropriate responses are brought to mitigate threats and vulnerabilities. Outputs of continuous monitoring are used by enterprise risk managers to make decisions that reflect the priorities established by leadership. Further referencing Sun Tzu, "If he sends reinforcements everywhere, he will everywhere be weak."[5] Effective cyberdefense necessitates strong prioritization and is the foundation for preparing the organization to respond *inside* its own and its adversaries' OODA loop.

Defensive and resilience strategies that negate threat speed and optimize time

Views of cybertime, the technology lifecycle, and incident and threat data are presented logarithmically in Figure 13.1. Attacks are instantaneous and are generally completed before detection, which is far too late. This figure provides examples of activities that should be prioritized at specific recommended frequencies, with the color-coding designating an urgency rating to each. This

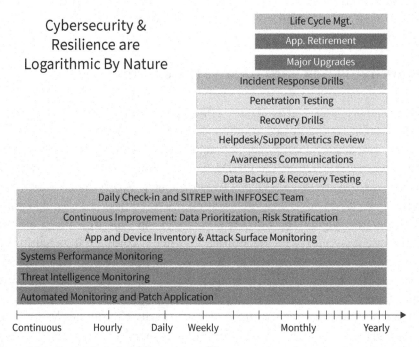

Figure 13.1 Tactics for prioritizing cyberresilience over time.

chart is best used as a starting point to assess operational readiness and to baseline new and existing cyberoperational strategies.

In our experience, most organizations are either quite close to this state of maturity or quite far away. Some organizations are doing some of it, but very few are doing all of it, and even fewer are doing all of it in a repeatable and reliable manner. More than anything else, dedicated personnel, focus, consistency, and cadence are key.

Stronger information technology

Establishment of cyberresiliency should be an intentional mix of proactive and reactive strategies. Starting with the proactive, cybersecurity isn't just, or even mostly about cyberdefense, it is about strong information technology (IT). The older an infrastructure, the more vulnerable it is to attacks and the more expensive it is to maintain. Organizations that wait too long to modernize IT not only greatly increase their cyberrisk but also may increase their liability as failure to adopt stronger and more resilient technologies may be viewed negatively by cyberinsurers and courts.[6] Key technology strategies must include: identification of organizational protection needs; security by design prior to implementation; minimization of potential cyberattack surface; detailed operational and investment plans to keep infrastructure current; daily patching; redundancy of data and systems; solid record keeping; regular testing of all data and systems backup and recovery processes; proactive external audit and testing, as well as a quality feed and daily review of current and ongoing threat intelligence.

Engage in organizational risk management

Adopting strategies that acknowledge time as the denominator is the key to maximizing cyberdefense. This begins with an organizational risk management approach such as Managing Information Security Risk (NIST 800-39) or the NIST Cybersecurity Framework ID.RM control. A key assumption is that organizational leadership will devote *frequent* and *routine* amounts of time to risk management activities. The frequency and amount of time applied to risk management activities drives the organizational sense of urgency regarding risk management and is the critical factor in the effectiveness of the approach. Time devoted to this activity is an expression of an organization's *risk tolerance*. NIST has recently updated the Risk Management Framework

(NIST SP800-37r2) with a special focus on preparation activities necessary to ensure that an organization is capable of conducting risk management.[7]

Prioritize and protect the most critical data

Minimizing an attack surface creates value beyond the reduction of endpoints as it drives data prioritization. Regardless of industry type, all organizations have a stratum of risk that is inherent in the data that they collect, utilize, share, and report, although most try to protect everything as though it were of equal value. Data should be stored, managed, and protected based upon the risk of loss or exposure of that data. The previously discussed EU General Data Protection Regulation (GDPR) may ultimately become the minimum criteria for all data privacy regulation. Cybersecurity and privacy must be a cornerstone of the business culture. Data that carry lower risk should be managed quite differently than critical data; and, as a result, prove less expensive to manage both in time and in money. Fort Knox isn't full of copper pennies; it is full of gold bars. Lastly, stratified data protection also enables advanced cyberresilience strategies such as using decoy data and systems to divert, fool, and possibly trap a cyber adversary.[8]

Caveat emptor when selecting cyber tools and partners

A dizzying array of commercial tools and solutions can be brought to bear to address the increasing cyberthreat. In fact, a Periodic Table of 140 cybersecurity firms that represent this market has been ingeniously composed.[9] The leading and emerging domains are secure communications, predictive intelligence, deception security, autonomous systems, IoT security, mobile security, cyberinsurance, network and endpoint security, and anti-fraud security. It is beyond the scope of this writing to consider these solutions in detail and important to note that the right collection of tools will only be effective when applied along with the right people and processes. Tools alone will not ensure security and resiliency. This cannot be overstated! Furthermore, the buyer must be diligent and beware, not only of any given partner, technology, or tool but also of the complexity of integrating multiple partners and new toolsets. Complexity, and its associated risks, can grow far more quickly than most expect and is in itself risky. That said, significant improvements in security posture can be achieved through application of innovative solutions, and smart shoppers can benefit when they are armed with knowledge of their specific protection needs and risk tolerances.

Social esprit de corps: Creating a functioning culture of cyberawareness

There has been extensive treatment of the benefit of establishing a cyber-aware culture in the workplace and the lay press, as well as in the technology and services advertising media. Although most of these articles and reports do a fair job admiring the problem, compliance-driven approaches such as formal training, signage, computer banners, and other methods that do raise awareness fall well short of accomplishing true cultural change. Furthermore, most cyberawareness is driven by standards and policies that do not evolve adequately in cybertime. In fact, the best place to study real cultural change is to visit an organization that has fallen victim to a major cyberattack. Not only is the change palpable and measurable, but those who have lived through the experience will relate how deep and profound course changes must be. In fact, transformation to a truly cyberaware culture is no less than a revolution in how an organization makes fundamental business decisions. Cybersecurity is not solely an IT issue, a risk management issue, a legal liability issue, or an executive leadership issue; it is now a fundamental environmental aspect of any business that uses, exploits, or depends upon technology. The future is now, and cybersecurity will be judged as a basic business competency along with fiscal responsibility, regulatory compliance, and all other competencies in the firmament of responsible businesses.

Putting cybersecurity in the C-suite and workforce

Organizations that respond in cybertime will be led by executives who are closely involved in managing the risk of cyberthreats.[10] The C-suite should ensure that organizational policies, actions, and attitudes do not promote a culture of "burying head(s) in the sand" or noncompliance with mitigations to cyber threats. These executives must keep the responsibility in the C-suite for protecting the organization from cyberthreats and must ensure that the organization is empowered with relevant and actionable threat information. They must also ensure that the processes for managing this information in the context of other business risks are prioritized. The goal of these efforts is to ensure decisive action and effective mitigations, as well as to understand cyberrisks based on the impact to the organization's goals.

The estimated shortage of cybersecurity workers is expected to be 1.8 million by 2022.[11] Prioritizing this already scarce resource further ensures that organizations are able to protect what is most important. Furthermore, it should be a strategic objective to promote cyberskills where they can have the biggest impact on an organization. Presidential Executive Order 13800 directs the Secretary of Commerce and the Secretary of Homeland Security to "jointly assess the scope and sufficiency of efforts to educate and train the American cybersecurity workforce" and to produce a report to the President "with findings and recommendations regarding how to support the growth and sustainment of the Nation's cybersecurity workforce."[12] All organizations should be doing the same but even faster.

As recently as the 1980s, biology was taught at the university level as a qualitative science not as a computer science as it is now taught. Advances in genetics, genomics, molecular imaging, and so many other technologies have transformed the basics of biological sciences. The same is happening in many other domains and necessitates a fundamentally different workforce composition. Cybersecurity and privacy skills are not only required in most positions but are necessary to ensure that these concerns are managed as part of an organizational risk-management process. It's too late in the game to have the chief information security officer (CISO) manage whether or not a new service requires privacy data from patients to be effective. Complicating this is that many of today's corporate and government leaders still view cyberthreats and good cyberhygiene as new and nonintuitive. The growing millennial workforce brings a fundamentally different view of technology and privacy, and companies should be incorporating this familiarity throughout an organization to build and reinforce security-aware corporate cultures.

In conclusion, the adversary is moving at unprecedented speed and organizations must be in position. We have presented a number of areas of focus:

(1) Be able to respond in cybertime to threats and vulnerabilities
(2) Manage cyberrisks in accordance with a methodology that results in priorities
(3) Select tools that meet your needs (know your requirements)
(4) The organization matters. Foster a cybersecurity culture that is based on your risk tolerance

Health care must commit to putting patient safety first. In the domain of cyberthreat, this means staying ahead of adversaries in real time.

References

1. Microsoft. Security Bulletins. Accessed May 2019. https://docs.microsoft.com/en-us/security-updates/

2. Gordon WJ, A Fairhall, and A Landman. Threats to Information Security—Public Health Implications. *New England Journal of Medicine* 2017. 377(8):707–709.

3. Feloni R, and A Pelisson. A Retired Marine and Elite Fighter Pilot Breaks Down the OODA Loop, the Military Decision-Making Process that Guides "Every Single Thing" in Life. *Business Insider* 2017, August 17.

4. National Institute of Standards and Technology. Information Security Continuous Monitoring (ISCM) for Federal Information Systems and Organizations. 2011, September. NIST Special Publication 800-137.

5. Sun Tzu. The Art of War. Accessed May 2018. http://classics.mit.edu/Tzu/artwar.html

6. National Association of Insurance Commissioners. Data, Innovation and Cyber. 2019, September 18. Accessed January 2020. https://content.naic.org/cipr_topics/topic_data_innovation_and_cyber.htm

7. National Institute of Standards and Technology. Risk Management Framework for Information Systems and Organizations: A System Life Cycle Approach for Security and Privacy. 2018, May 9. Accessed May 2019. https://csrc.nist.gov/CSRC/media/Publications/sp/800-37/rev-2/draft/documents/sp800-37r2-discussion-draft.pdf

8. Voris J et al. Bait and Snitch: Defending Computer Systems with Decoys. Columbia University Department of Computer Science online source. Accessed January 2020. http://nsl.cs.columbia.edu/papers/2012/baitsnitch.cip12.pdf

9. CBINsights. The Periodic Table of Cybersecurity Startups. 2017, March 23. Accessed January 2020. https://www.cbinsights.com/research/periodic-table-cybersecurity-startups/

10. PWC. How Businesses Can Build the Resilience Needed to Withstand Disruptive Cyberattacks. 2018. Accessed January 2020. https://www.pwc.com/us/en/cybersecurity/assets/pwc-2018-gsiss-strengthening-digital-society-against-cyber-shocks.pdf

11. Kawamoto D. Cybersecurity Faces 1.8 Million Worker Shortfall by 2022. *Dark Reading*. 2017, June 7.

12. Whitehouse.gov. Presidential Executive Order on Strengthening the Cybersecurity of Federal Networks and Critical Infrastructure. 2017, May 11.

14

Quantifying Cyberthreat for Patients, Providers, and Institutions

Medicine and math

Medicine has an uneasy relationship with math. On one hand, epidemiology, the study of the incidence, distribution, and other quantitative aspects of health and disease, is steeped in mathematics. Conversely, people are not statistics and the numbers may be less than helpful to any given patient and/ or clinician during a clinical encounter. For example, I have been managing a relatively low-incidence, or rare, form of kidney cancer for more than 15 years. At one point, my oncologist was following three other patients with the exact same tumor pathology. All of them were over 70 years of age at first presentation of disease, African American, and all are clinically obese. I, on the other hand, was diagnosed at 38 years of age, am of Caucasian descent, and have a relatively low body mass index. So much for standard distributions of disease . . .

The highest level of interaction is at the population level, where things are measured, assumed, and reported to be true with a certain level of precision. For example, it is estimated by one source that 1 out of 10,000 people will have an adverse reaction to general anesthesia with a possible error of up to 70%, which means up to 1.7 people per 10,000 may have an adverse reaction.[1] One study examined perioperative anaphylaxis, collected and reviewed 266 reports of Grades 3–5 anaphylaxis over 1 year from all National Health Service (NHS) hospitals in the United Kingdom. Out of these 266 cases, there were 10 deaths and 40 cardiac arrests. So, the risk of an event was 1 out of 10,000, and the risk of death from that event was approximately 4%. These numbers show that, overall, general anesthesia is safe, but how is "safe" determined? Without jumping too deeply into statistics, the rule of three is often utilized. Simply put, the rule of three means that you need three times as many subjects to observe an event when you assume that the adverse event of interest does not normally occur in the absence of the medication.[2] Specifically, if a new medication caused serious adverse reactions in 1 in 1,000 cases, you need to study

Digital Health. Eric D. Perakslis and Martin Stanley, Oxford University Press (2021). © Oxford University Press.
DOI: 10.1093/oso/9780197503133.003.0014

3,000 subjects (rule of three) in order to have a 95% chance of detecting even one case. Applying this math to the above example on general anesthesia, the stated 1-in-10,000 risk can only be considered true with a 95% confidence interval if the population studied is 65,000 cases or larger. Lastly, in consideration of exactly what "rare" means, a rule of thumb is that rare events are those that occur between 1/1,000 and 1/10,000 patients with very rare events occurring less frequently than 1/10,000.

Of course, numbers do not tell nearly all of the story when it comes to medicine, given that the severity of the event matters. An extremely rare but catastrophic event, such as death, will likely be managed differently than a more common event such as mild headache. This particular situation can cause an interesting dilemma for biomedical product developers and regulators. At one point in my career while working in drug discovery and development, my company detected a very rare but potentially fatal adverse event associated with a drug. The company contacted the Food and Drug Administration (FDA) and suggested that a box warning be placed on the product even though the event was rare. Surprisingly, the agency pushed back on the warning. Their reasoning was that the drug was the only available treatment option for a serious disorder, and they were concerned that the warning would deter use, leaving no desirable treatment options for those in need. It was fascinating and unexpected to witness a situation where a drug sponsor was arguing for a safety warning on one of their products while the regulators argued against. In the end, a carefully worded warning and specific additional guidance for doctors was issued. At the heart of the compromise was the concern that our company felt compelled to communicate this rare risk and certainly was likely to be liable for not communicating the risk if/when a patient suffered an instance of the event.

The last, but by no means the least, important perspective is that of the individual who suffers the rare or very rare events. The anesthesia adverse event statistics in the United States align reasonably well with those previously cited in the NHS example, with an anesthesia death rate of roughly one out of 1.1 million cases. Given that there are approximately 40 million surgeries per year in the United States, this means that roughly 36 people per year are lost to these events.[5] The good news is that any one of us has a relatively low risk of dying during general anesthesia. The bad news is that these statistics are not at all comforting to the families of the 36 people who are lost annually. Medicine will never be perfect, and practitioners know this better than anyone given that, eventually, they will be confronted with one of these horrible types of events. When that happens, the statistics are no comfort.

In the digital age, this phenomenon can be amplified in challenging ways. Take the antivaccine movement. If one disregards misinformation, it is still quite possible to bump into the family of a child who actually did have a severe adverse reaction to a vaccine, as they rarely do occur. As discussed in the chapter on medical misinformation, messages are easily amplified and distorted in the digital age and medicine plays a part. Despite the best intentions, shouting, "vaccines are safe!" at the anti-vaxxers may be feeding the debate, given that it may ignore those in the crowd who have experienced the rare trauma. The truth, of course, is that vaccines are *usually* safe. For those with concerns who want to know the exact numbers, the data should be shared and discussed rationally, despite those who feel that sharing numbers weakens the case by exposing the specific numbers and underlying studies to criticism.

Determining the incidence of cyberevents in health care

Although difficult to study directly, the size and scale of healthcare hacks indicates their occurrence to be quite high at the population level, given that most views taken from various sources point to extremely high prevalence. Examples include a study using data collected by the Office for Civil Rights, Department of Health and Human Services (HHS), which concluded that over half of the population in the United States might have been affected by security breaches since October 2009.[6] A study in the HIPAA journal shows that reported healthcare data breaches per year grew from 18 in 2009 to 365 in 2018; it also revealed that the average breach size is more than 2,000 affected records but with instances as high as more than 400,000 records per breach.[7] However, because this study only included data through 2018, the incidence reported by mid-2019 was already at 31,000,000 records, more than double the full year 2018 value, with 88% of the breaches known to be caused by hacking.[8] The data are clear that the incidence is high and growing rapidly, with factors pointing toward health care as the most highly targeted and profitable sector for cybercrime.[9]

Examining these numbers, with a public-health eye, it is interesting to consider the best ways to apply epidemiological vernacular to healthcare breach incidence. According to the Centers for Disease Control and Prevention (CDC), a common definition for an epidemic is an increase, often sudden, in the number of cases of a disease above what is normally expected in that population in that area.[10] This requires an understanding of what is "normally expected," that is, the endemic amount of disease in a given population. So, depending on one's chosen perspective, given that more than half the population of the United States has likely been the victim of a healthcare data breach, we are either in the 10th year of an outbreak that has clearly reached epidemic proportions, or healthcare cybercrime is now hyperendemic and affecting more than 50% of our population.

Within this theme of comparing cybercrime to disease incidence, there are significant limitations as are discussed in detail at the end of this chapter. That said, the precision and accuracy of the data associated with a specific breach is certainly better than aggregated statistics from across data breaches where underlying differences in the data could cause misinterpretations. Using specific reports, far more precise comparisons can be made, as shown in the examples that follow.

These days, large healthcare hacks barely make the headlines and, unfortunately, this indicates a potential level of desensitization. We would be unwise, however, to not put these hacks into an epidemiological context, given that the impacts must be understood. Otherwise, this lucrative avenue of crime will continue to grow at an even greater pace. According to the previously referenced Protenus breach barometer, there were 32 million records breached in the first half of 2019, and 88% of these breaches, 28.2 million, were caused by hacking. This indicates the incidence of cybercrime in the first half of 2019 to be almost exactly equivalent to the number of people living with type 2 diabetes in the United States.[11] The number of individuals affected by the Banner Health hack of 2016 was greater than the number of people living with type 1 diabetes in the United States. The number of records exposed during the 21st Century Oncology Hack of 2016 was 20% greater than the average number of patients who are diagnosed with cancer annually.[12] The Excellus Health Plan breach of 2015 exposed 10,000,000 records, roughly equivalent to twice the number of people in the United States living with congestive heart failure. The number of records exposed by the Anthem data breach of 2015 is more than twice the worst estimates of annual influenza occurrence published by the CDC. Need we go on? Once these data are placed into this type of healthcare-specific context, the ability for an adversary to have an adverse impact on a large population is difficult to ignore.

Looking into the prevalence of medical device intrusions and tampering, it is difficult to know exactly where things stand, but the evidence points to a high prevalence of hidden or occult disease. Most studies to date have focused upon the vulnerability of various types of medical devices but not on incidence. This leaves us in the uncomfortable spot of knowing that these devices are highly vulnerable and that once compromised they are seldom ever detected, but we are left with little visibility into the likelihood. That said, the part of the field that is trying to keep pace is focused on understanding the potential vulnerability of individual or specific classes of medical devices. For example, because of their direct connectivity and functionality, pacemakers, infusion pumps, and diagnostic equipment, such as MRI machines, are considered to carry the highest levels of danger to humans if hacked or misused.[14] It is the misuse of such systems that is of greatest concern for several reasons not the least of which is altering the system's integrity. First, an attack that disables a device usually renders the device inoperable, which leads to the device being taken out of service, thereby eliminating the possibility of the device causing harm. Second, attacks that steal data similarly do not necessarily impede the primary purpose of the device, unless the hacks are focused on altering the functionality or disabling the device. Misuse, however, is a very different level of risk, because it can be insidious and go on undetected for an extended period of time. For example, consider a hypothetical hack that increases the rate of infusion on every infusion pump on a particular hospital network by one third. The immediate response would likely be to suspect user error. It also might take quite a while for the various teams involved to realize that what they are noticing is not an isolated incident. Depending on the patient and drug being infused, as well as the quantity in the intravenous (IV) bag, the effects could range from minor to disastrous across a diverse collection of patients, drugs, and infirmities.

Another important consideration is that many consider hospital data networks to be medical devices from the standpoint of risk, because hospital networks provide an important pathway for essential communication, such as between bedside instrument alerts and a nursing station. This is a particularly important issue when thinking through elements of digital health that involve home monitoring or data exchange. If real-time data is being transmitted from a device to a healthcare institution through a home network, then the network itself must be considered an essential component of the digital device simply because outages may have serious consequences. These types of interdependency remind us that, in the connected Internet-of-Things world, what we are also connecting is risk, which magnifies as the area of connectivity grows.

Impact of cyberevents in health care

One of the most important fundamentals of understanding risk is determining impact. As discussed in the previous chapters, a privacy impact does not necessarily cause harm in itself but the result of that loss of privacy may. Specifically, if personal financial information is stolen from a hospital, actual harm to any given victim may not be realized until that stolen information is used to do something, such as open a bogus retail credit card account. In this hypothetical case, the resulting harm could be financial liability and/or credit rating damage due to bogus financial transaction data. With respect to health care, it is clear that much of the potential harm of healthcare data breaches lies in cyber and identity theft. According to a study in the *Annals of Internal Medicine* from September 2019 that studied the specifics of data lost/stolen in healthcare data breaches, a total of 513 breaches (35%) compromised service or financial information. Among them, 186 breaches (13%) affecting 49 million patients (29%) compromised sensitive financial information (i.e., credit cards or banking accounts), and a total of 944 breaches (65%) compromised the medical or clinical information of 48 million patients (28%).[15]

Another impact of stolen health and personal information is when criminals use that data to procure health care, prescriptions, and medical equipment. According to Stephanie Armour in a *Wall Street Journal* piece, "Adding insult to injury, a victim often can't fully examine his own records because the thief's health data, now folded into his, are protected by medical-privacy laws. And hospitals sometimes continue to hound victims for payments they didn't incur."[17] This type of crime is not only exceptionally troublesome and frustrating for the victims, there is a no time limit for the damage. When a hacked institution offers free identity monitoring for a year following a breach disclosure, the remedy is limited by the fact that the data may be used years after the original breach. Further, in cases where breeched organizations claim little liability based upon the assertion that the compromised data was encrypted, there is really no way to know how far in the future an encryption methodology will remain secure. At any time, a method may be developed that nullifies the effectiveness of any given encryption technology and stolen data can hypothetically exist forever on the dark web, in the hordes of cybercriminals and/or many other similar places.

Patient safety

According to the ECRI Institute, a nonprofit that has focused on the safety of medical devices and clinical environments, the ability of hackers to exploit remote access to systems to disrupt healthcare operations was the number one patient safety risk on its 2019 annual list of Health Technology Hazards.[17] Other top hazards included improperly set ventilator arms, retention of surgical sponges, fall risks from overhead lift systems, mishandling of endoscopes after disinfection, and fluid seepage onto patients or equipment. What is most interesting about this particular list is that it is one of the first to place cybersecurity of medical devices directly into the context of other more traditional and well-known patient safety hazards. According to ECRI, the topic nomination and selection criteria include investigating incidents, testing of medical devices, observing operations, assessing hospital practices, literature reviews, and interviews with clinicians, clinical engineers, technology managers, purchasing staff, health systems administrators, and device suppliers. The factors weighted for final inclusion and ranking are diverse, covering many factors of risk, safety, and liability including severity, frequency, breadth, insidiousness, reputational impact, and preventability. Such a comprehensive set of factors clearly represents benefit-risk assessment at a level rarely applied by U.S. regulators to the safety assessment of medical devices, but it probably should be applied more frequently.

There also is a strong basis for the selection of remote access as the underlying key vulnerability. According to the Rapid7, a top cybersecurity firm, quarterly threat report released May 15, 2018, health care was the industry most targeted by cybercrime in the first quarter of 2018. The research found that the leading attack vectors in health care were remote access (e.g., suspicious logins), access attempts from disabled accounts, and account leaks, as well as phishing and ransomware.[18]

Other clear warnings of the risk of cyberthreat to health care come from the *Report On Improving Cybersecurity in the Health Care Industry*, published by HHS in 2017, which states, "The healthcare and public health sector is charged with keeping patients safe. "This includes physical and privacy related harms that may stem from a cybersecurity vulnerability or exploit . . . Such outcomes could have a profound impact on patient care and safety."[20] This report cited 23 patient safety risks but did not elaborate them qualitatively or quantitatively. The lack of quantitative evidence is one of the significant limitations of this study and, possibly, the reason that the impact of the report has been limited.

One of the major challenges in quantifying the effects of cybersecurity on patient risks is that root-cause analysis seldom considers engineering domains. If a machine malfunctions, the malfunction is noted, but the root cause of the malfunction is not identified. Although technology has been blended seamlessly into health care, it has not happened in a way in which the impacts and implications of technology are clear, transparent, and understandable. Add in patient confidentiality, the legal practices around liability, and low general technology literacy, and it becomes clear that the "black box" problem discussed in the sections on algorithms is not at all limited to algorithms. Rather, it is applicable to the devices themselves, increased complexity in the environment, and many other facets of healthcare digitization. The bottom line is that well-designed quantitative studies are essential to ensure patient safety.

Cyberwar and current events

One of the unique and most perilous aspects of the digitization of health care is the level of geopolitical threat as well as the diverse nature of these threats. Hospitals typically have not been targets of traditional shooting wars, although recent events in the Syrian conflicts have witnessed exactly this, and many institutions have no level of awareness or preparation for these types of risks. One recent example is Jon Riggi, Senior Advisor of Cybersecurity and Risk Advisory Services at the American Hospital Association discussing the increased risk of cyberattacks due to the recent escalating friction with Iran and how hospitals and health systems can protect themselves.[21] Mr. Riggi categorizes both direct and indirect threats. During times of conflict or increased international tension, the likelihood of state-sponsored cyberattacks, such as WannaCry ransomware, increases sharply. There is also an increased likelihood of spikes in cybercrime that can be compared to the types of looting that are seen during physical disaster scenarios. Motivations for both include intimidation, reputational damage, and simple theft. These threats are not hyperacute for institutions that have solid cybersecurity capabilities but are very dangerous for the unprepared. What may be less obvious and easy to understand are the more indirect threats, such as cyberattacks against critical infrastructure, for example, public utilities. Attacks on the power grid, communications grid, water utilities, and sewage treatment plants could all cause unanticipated cascading effects for which it might be difficult to plan. These types of attacks also have the potential to cause civil unrest in affected areas that not only could threaten healthcare workers and facilities directly but also increase patient burden.

One recent example are the warnings issued after the killing of Iran's top military commander Qassem Soleimani in a U.S. drone attack in late 2019. According to the *Financial Times* on January 5, 2020, government officials warned of cyberattacks that could target corporate and municipal IT systems, transit, logistics, military, and healthcare systems.[22] The purpose of these types of attacks is disruption and intimidation. According to John Hultquist, a cybersecurity expert at Fireye, "the purpose of such attacks is to show the American people that they can reach out and touch us." Again, quantification of these threats is not typically shared due to the sensitive nature of the threat intelligence, but we know they exist.

Cyberthreat is a gateway

Lastly, it is important to understand that in the digital world cyberthreat is not only itself a threat, but it is also a gateway to most of the 10 Toxicities. Think about the doors and windows to your home. They serve the purpose of letting you enter and exit, but they also keep bad weather out, insulate you against the elements, protect you from unauthorized intrusion that could lead to theft, vandalism, arson, and even personal liability. These are not crimes of doors and windows, they are crimes of unwanted access, intrusion, and violation. This is the importance of cyberprotections in modern digital health; they are the first and last line of defense against almost all of the things that can go wrong. Further, the striking statistics surrounding hacks and data breaches must forewarn us that, for the most part, our doors and windows are wide open, and patients are not being protected. If this were the case for physical security within our health system, patients and providers would be up in arms shouting for change. If the vulnerabilities of Internet-connected health care were better understood, they would be demanding improved safety.

Limitations of these data and the scope of our research

There are significant limitations to quantitative analysis of this type given limitations of the available data sources. Examples of limitations include inadequately annotated and/or qualified source data, lack of detail, and lack of downloadable or verifiable source data. All these gaps are usual in cybersecurity, given that for many reasons intimate details of exploits often are not shared. First, there may be ongoing liability litigation around an event that requires evidence confidentiality. Second, threat data is often also considered sensitive, because the more an adversary understands the intelligence, tactics, and strategies of who they wish to attack, the more targeted those attacks can be. Lastly, full information regarding an exploit may not be understood until well after the incident has been remediated. This is truly "Art of War" stuff, and the primary difference between cyberthreat and many other medical risk factors is the simple unavoidable truth that there is an adversary that must be considered.

References

1. Harper NJN et al. Anaesthesia, Surgery, and Life-Threatening Allergic Reactions: Epidemiology and Clinical Features of Perioperative Anaphylaxis in the 6th National Audit Project (NAP6). *British Journal of Anaesthesia* 2018. 121(1):159–171.
2. Onakpuya I. Rare Adverse Events in Clinical Trials: Understanding the Rule of Three. BMJ Blog. 2017, November 14. https://blogs.bmj.com/bmjebmspotlight/2017/11/14/rare-adverse-events-clinical-trials-understanding-rule-three/
3. Chan EW, KQ Liu, CS Chui, CW Sing, LY Wong, and IC Wong. Adverse Drug Reactions—Examples of Detection of Rare Events Using Databases. *British Journal of Clinical Pharmacology* 2015. 80(4):855–861.
4. Li G, M Warner, BH Lang, L Huang, and LS Sun. Epidemiology of Anesthesia-Related Mortality in the United States, 1999–2005. *Anesthesiology* 2009. 110(4):759–765.
5. CDC. Ambulatory Surgery Data from Hospitals and Ambulatory Surgery Centers USA: 2010. 2017, February 28. Accessed January 2020. https://www.cdc.gov/nchs/data/nhsr/nhsr102.pdf
6. Koczkodaj WW, J Masiak, M Mazurek, D Strzałka, and PF Zabrodskii. Massive Health Record Breaches Evidenced by the Office for Civil Rights Data. *Iranian Journal of Public Health* 2019. 48(2):278–288.
7. HIPAA Journal. Healthcare Data Breach Statistics. Accessed January 2020. https://www.hipaajournal.com/healthcare-data-breach-statistics/
8. Davis J. 32 Million Patient Records Breached in the First Half of 2019, 88% Caused by Hacking. *Health IT Security*. 2019, August 1.
9. CSO Online. Healthcare Ailing in Cyber War. https://www.csoonline.com/article/3215968/healthcare-ailing-in-cyber-war.html
10. CDC. Introduction to Epidemiology. 2012, May 18. Accessed January 2020. https://www.cdc.gov/csels/dsepd/ss1978/lesson1/section11.html
11. CDC. Type 2 Diabetes. 2019, May 30. Accessed January 2020. https://www.cdc.gov/diabetes/basics/type2.html
12. Cancer.gov. Cancer Statistics. National Cancer Institute. 2018, April 27. Accessed January 2020. https://www.cancer.gov/about-cancer/understanding/statistics
13. CDC. Disease Burden of Influenza. 2020, January 10. Accessed January 2020. https://www.cdc.gov/flu/about/burden/index.html
14. Alpine Security. Most Dangerous Hacked Medical Devices. Accessed January 2020. https://www.alpinesecurity.com/blog/most-dangerous-hacked-medical-devices
15. Jiang JX, and G Bai. Types of Information Compromised in Breaches of Protected Health Information [published online ahead of print, 2019, September 24]. *Annals of Internal Medicine* 2019. doi: 10.7326/M19-1759.
16. Armour S. How Identity Theft Sticks You with Hospital Bills. *Wall Street Journal*. 2015, August 7.
17. ECRI Institute. 2019 Top Ten Health Technology Hazards. 2018. Accessed January 2020. https://www.ecri.org/Resources/Whitepapers_and_reports/Haz_19.pdf
18. Donovan F. Cyberattacks Exploiting Weaknesses in Healthcare Data Security. *Health IT Security*. 2018, May 15.
19. Donovan F. SamSam Ransomware Attackers Target Healthcare Providers. *Health IT Security*. 2018, April 12.
20. HHS Healthcare Industry Cybersecurity Task Force. Report on Improving Cybersecurity in the Healthcare Industry. 2017, June. Accessed January 2020. https://www.phe.gov/Preparedness/planning/CyberTF/Documents/report2017.pdf

21. American Hospital Association. Cybersecurity Threat Assessment. AHA Podcast. Accessed January 2020. https://www.aha.org/advancing-health-podcast/2020-01-17-cybersecurity-threat-assessment

22. Murphy H. US on High Alert for Iran-backed Cyberattacks. *Financial Times*. 2020, January 5.

15

Case Studies

Notable Healthcare Hacks and Lessons Learned

Boston Children's Hospital and hacktivism

"In real-world war, combatants typically don't attack hospitals . . . hackers have no such scruples . . . We're attacked about every 7 seconds, 24 hours a day," said John Halamka MD, who was chief information officer (CIO) of the Boston hospital Beth Israel Deaconess at the time, speaking on a panel at a national meeting. "And the strikes come from everywhere: It's hacktivists, organized crime, cyberterrorists and MIT students."[1] From a historical perspective, Dr Halamka was correct, and the point cannot be overstated, given that health care has been late to recognize or take action against cyberthreat. Regrettably, in 2018–2019, the core statement that hospitals are typically not attacked in conventional war was also proven false with horrific bombings of hospitals in Syria and other conflict zones.[2] Unfortunately, war is different now than it has ever been and terror, intimidation, and horrific acts without fear of retribution have almost become background noise. In 2019, healthcare cyberattacks were up 60% in the first nine months compared to 2018, and the variety of attacks, from ransomware to attacks on medical devices increased simultaneously.[3] These real-world examples are presented in hopes that resources can be prioritized and proactive measures enacted for medical cybersecurity.

Shortly after starting my time as Executive Director of the Center for Biomedical Informatics at Harvard Medical School, I was asked to join several Harvard hospital-based working groups on cybersecurity. It was late 2013, and 40 million holiday shoppers at Target retail stores had just had their debit and credit card numbers stolen.[4] There were also high-profile hacks at *The New York Times*, JP Morgan, the U.S. Federal Reserve, the National Aeronautics and Space Administration (NASA), the U.S. Energy Department, Facebook, and Apple, but health care had been left essentially untouched. Having most recently served as the CIO and Chief Scientist (Informatics) at the FDA, I had studied and worked on what the federal government knew to be a rapidly increasing level of cyberthreat. This knowledge, coupled with my

Digital Health. Eric D. Perakslis and Martin Stanley, Oxford University Press (2021). © Oxford University Press.
DOI: 10.1093/oso/9780197503133.003.0015

background in healthcare technology and medical safety, led me to sense that things were going to change quickly in health care.

As a fledgling academic, I decided to publish a piece on healthcare cybersecurity intended to warn and wake up the healthcare industry. I submitted a prospective article to the *New England Journal of Medicine* in February of 2014. The piece was rejected, but I was invited to revise and resubmit, which I did the following April. Later that month, Boston Children's Hospital (BCH) was the victim of a major distributed denial of service (DDOS) cyberattack. Dan Nigrin MD, CIO of BCH later detailed the events of the cyberattack for the *New England Journal of Medicine*:

> The attack began with a warning message on Twitter, attributed to Anonymous, about a highly publicized child-custody case, in which a patient with a complex diagnostic presentation was eventually taken into custody by Massachusetts protective services. The message threatened the hospital with retaliation if we did not comply with certain demands, including taking disciplinary action against specific clinicians and returning the child to her parents (despite the fact that she was no longer at the hospital). The initial attack consisted of posting the home and work addresses, phone numbers, and e-mail addresses of some of the people involved in the case (a tactic called "doxing"). The hackers also posted technical information about the hospital's public-facing website, suggesting that it might become a target.

Several weeks later, the hospital began to experience a low-level "distributed denial of service" (DDoS) attack directed against its external website. A DDoS attack is meant to make a website or resource unavailable for its intended use by saturating it with so many communication requests that it can no longer respond to legitimate ones; such attacks may ultimately overload the server, the organization's bandwidth, or both. Over a period of a week, the volume of the DDoS attack was sequentially increased, and at its peak there was enough malicious inbound network traffic to significantly slow legitimate inbound and outbound traffic.[5] The attack went on to affect other organizations that used the same Internet service provider (ISP) as BCH. There were also other forms of attacks intended to penetrate the firewalls of BCH, such as spear-fishing e-mails. In the end, no patients were harmed, but there were significant and prolonged disruptions of hospital operations as well as a wake-up call to which the healthcare industry has been slow to respond.

Interestingly, some of the most notable and important parts of this story are not the technical details. First, the threat of hacktivism, the utilization of cyberattacks to bring attention to a cause, became a recognized threat to health care. Previously, higher profile hacktivism attacks were political/governmental in nature, such as attacks by this same group, Anonymous, during the Arab Spring movements of 2010. Health care and other industries had not yet recognized the threat and, surely, institutions such as children's hospitals, which have a reputation as institutions of public good, did not see these types of threats coming. Another key piece was the interconnectivity of systems. If you have ever taken a look at the thick stream of wires emanating from the electric breaker box in your home, you have noticed that it is not obvious or even easy to discern where those wires go. Now think about the network wires in major institutions of many floors, many buildings, and decades of new construction and remodeling. It should then be easy to imagine how cyberattacks could spread quickly and be quite difficult to follow, as well as how challenging it would be to determine all of the impacts. Similarly, another key point, which Dr Nigrin also describes in his *New England Journal of Medicine* piece, is how difficult it can be to realize an institution's dependency on e-mail. During a significant cyberattack, even if e-mail is not affected or directly a target, the e-mail system can be a route of propagation that often needs to be shut down temporarily as malware and other attack vectors propagate rapidly and extensively via e-mail. When actions such as shutting down the e-mail system are taken there are unintended consequences. For example, the operations at many organizations depend upon automated e-mail messages and alerts. When those go down, alerts and automation stop. In the end, the BCH response led by Dan Nigrin and his team was effective and exceptional. The perpetrator was found, convicted, and sentenced to 10 years in jail.[7] The events served as a wake-up for health care that change was coming and that the digitization of health records and other processes carried significant new threats that would need to be addressed.

Several months after the attacks were disclosed and the effects covered extensively in the news media, I received an acceptance notice from the *New England Journal of Medicine* on my "Cybersecurity in Healthcare" piece. It was published in July of 2014 along with Dan Nigrin's detailed account of the attack on his hospital.[8] I was honored to publish alongside Dr Nigrin and amused that he has joked that I hacked his hospital just so I could get my piece into the *New England Journal of Medicine*. The piece now serves as a baseline for many articles and opinions on cybersecurity, and although many still did not buy into the level of imminent threat and coming attacks at that time, most in the industry now understand. That said, the level of understanding remains less than what is needed; although the threats to hospitals are far better understood, the corresponding threats to small clinics, doctor's offices, connected medical devices, healthcare digital tools, and many other potential targets are still not receiving the urgency, attention, or action that is warranted.

A wave of ransomware attacks

Ransomware is a form of cyberattack that essentially renders computer systems unavailable until ransom is paid to the attacker. The most common story of the origin of ransomware is that it originated in 1989 when Harvard-educated biologist Joseph L. Popp sent 20,000 compromised diskettes named "AIDS Information—Introductory Diskettes" to attendees of the internal AIDS conference organized by the World Health Organization. The Trojan horse worked by encrypting the file names on the victims' computers and hiding directories. The victims were asked to pay $189 to PC Cyborg Corp. care of a mailbox in Panama.[9] Generally speaking, the potential business impacts of ransomware are loss or destruction of crucial information and systems, as well as business downtime, lost productivity, lingering disruption, and damage to systems, data, files and reputations.

Ransomware has proven to be a highly profitable form of cybercrime; some consider it the most profitable form of malware. This is true for several reasons. First of all, ransomware can be used to target large legacy infrastructures where cyberprotections such as antimalware are difficult to keep fully up to date. This means that older malicious code that is relatively well known can still be used, thus avoiding the need for novel attack software. Backup and recovery processes within these outdated systems are also usually substandard, making it impossible for an enterprise to restore its own systems and data. Because large companies and government infrastructures often are made up of such dated computing infrastructure, and because they are likely to pay ransom, ransomware attacks often target these types of victims as opposed to spreading code across the Internet in random fashion.

Hospitals and healthcare facilities are ideal candidates for ransomware not only because many have complex computer systems that are easy to target, but also because loss of system function can be an urgent life-threatening matter. Even if critical systems are properly protected, losing medical record data forever would have significant impact on any facility and its patients. The effects of these attacks have been devastating. The threat has risen steadily since the early 2000s and many of the potential scenarios of ransomware in health care have played out. In fact, 2015 witnessed significant enough growth that the FBI issued a warning urging hospitals to take the threat seriously. The warning also urged affected organizations to not pay ransom, claiming,

Paying a ransom doesn't guarantee an organization that it will get its data back—we've seen cases where organizations never got a decryption key after having paid the ransom. Paying a ransom not only emboldens current cyber criminals to target more organizations, it also offers an incentive for other criminals to get involved in this type of illegal activity. And finally, by paying a ransom, an organization might inadvertently be funding other illicit activity associated with criminals.[10]

Further, the warning goes on to remind that basic cyberhygiene as well as properly designed and frequently tested backup and recovery controls offer the ounce of protection that may be enough to protect some institutions.

As of the time of this writing, ransomware incidence continues to rise and there appears to be at least one clear occurrence of any and all potential harms. According to the American Medical Association (AMA), 83% of physicians work in organizations that have experienced at least one cyberattack.[11] Individual case studies are striking. Examples of permanent clinic closures in 2019 include Wood Ranch Medical, a clinic in Simi Valley, California, that suffered a ransomware attack, and announced its closure citing, "damage to our computer system was such that we are unable to recover the data stored there and, with our backup system encrypted as well, we cannot rebuild our medical records."[12] A similar situation led to the closure of Brookside ENT and Hearing Center, based in Battle Creek, Michigan. These are far from isolated or rare incidents. In fact, incidents have become so common that they seldom make a dent in the 24-hour news cycle. Instead, these attacks are now being tabulated and communicated en masse. One such report in *Becker's Hospital Review* listed "15 Notable Ransomware Attacks on Healthcare Providers in 2019."[13] The list demonstrates no geographical or other form of preference or focus. Clinics large and small were targeted across the United States and impacts ranged from data breaches to altered operations to the previously referenced clinic closures.

Clearly, this is a growing business concern for health care but what are the impacts on patient care and safety? The WannaCry attack on the National Health Service (NHS) of the United Kingdom in May of 2017 is known to have cost almost 100 million pounds and caused significant disruption to patient care, including the cancellation of some 19,000 appointments—including surgeries—and the disruption of IT systems for at least a third of all NHS hospitals.[14] Clearly these are massive impacts on care delivery. With respect to patient safety, methodologies for studying the impacts are just now being developed. In one postmortem of the WannaCry attacks, no increase in mortality was reported based upon comparisons to historical data, but the authors admit that these are the crudest of measures.[15]

Measurement of harms associated with cyberattacks can be especially complex because the effects can be nonlinear, that is, present difficulty in determining direct causality, and because data is fragmented across so many health systems. For example, according to KrebsonSecurity, "what isn't yet known is how WannaCry affected mortality rates among heart attack and stroke patients whose ambulances were diverted to other hospitals because of IT system outages related to the malware."[16]

A study by researchers at Vanderbilt University was one of the first to examine the lingering effects of healthcare hacks; it found that the emergency "time-to-electrocardiogram" increased as much as 2.7 minutes and 30-day acute myocardial infarction mortality increased as much as 0.36 percentage points during the three-year window following a breach.[17] Although this important study has limitations, such as not considering specific cybercontrols that may have been put in place following a cyberattack, the effects discussed assert important logic. Specifically, the study concludes that breach remediation efforts, such as taking systems offline for updates and upgrades, can be as dangerous as the attacks, citing discontinuities in data and care that can surface over a period of years following the cyberattack. Another important impact of the study should be increased thoughtfulness regarding technology in health care. Healthcare delivery is a long and complex set of physical processes and data/technology processes. A single perturbation could affect outcomes in infinite ways that are difficult or even impossible to measure. The impact of a single missed visit across a large population afflicted with a range of common to unusual disorders is simply not that easy to quantify. The same is true for a few missing data elements in a medical record, a late pathology report that arrives after a clinician visit, or a slot set of clinician notes. All of these and many other situations and permutations of situations will need to be studied if we are to understand fully the hazards of mixing health care and cyberspace.

For now, as long as it remains profitable, ransomware will remain a threat to health care. Those who are not taking things seriously are not only putting patients and clinicians at risk but also the financial well-being of their institution. According to a recent FICO survey, as of late 2018, nearly 70% of U.S. healthcare providers hadn't purchased cyberinsurance.[18] The reasons cited in the survey are potentially of even more concern, with healthcare executives split over whether they expect cyberthreats and data breaches to stay the same or increase in the coming year (of course, every metric shows they are rising). Further, across all industries, executives perceive that senior IT management (31%) poses the highest risk to their organizations, followed by system administrators, internal IT staff (20%), and everyday business users

(16%)! It is hard to perceive these findings as anything other than down-right depressing, given that this particular study reveals that most healthcare executives are ignorant to cyberrisk and those who are aware feel their own people add to the risk instead of decreasing it.

The WannaCry cyberattack

At the risk of sounding like I am bad luck, just as with the hacktivist attack on Boston Children's hospital, I also have a personal connection to the WannaCry cyberattack. On the morning of Friday, May 12, 2017, I was working at home serving as a reviewer for an article on cybersecurity for the *British Medical Journal* (BMJ). It was a solid piece, but I often struggle to help with articles written by experts in one field who are somewhat novice in another. Doctors with an interest in studying, working, and writing on cybersecurity are a good example of this. They often have an expertly exquisite view and situational awareness of clinical settings, but they can lack adequate background, practical experience, and understanding in engineering, information technology, and technical operations. That said, what they do have is the ability to speak with authority to their peers and that is priceless.

Shortly after submitting my review, I received a note back from the editor asking if I was aware of the ongoing cyberattack that was affecting the NHS that very morning. At the time I was not, but as the effects and associated turmoil quickly became public, it was not difficult to get up to speed as well as one could do without being on the ground and having firsthand intelligence on the event. At that time, it was clear that malware had locked computers and had blocked access to patient files in England's public hospitals.[19] It is very easy to underestimate the fear and even panic that this type of disruption can bring.

Per our discussions on earlier case studies, it can be impossible for work to continue when regular processes are disrupted. Think of the steps in baking a cake. Certain things must happen in specific order, and they involve access to multiple systems. Now, what to do once the dry ingredients are mixed, but the refrigerator door is jammed so you cannot get to the eggs? You borrow some eggs, but the mixer won't work, so you beat the mixture by hand. You finally get the batter ready, but the oven will only hold temperature at 200 degrees or at 500 degrees, and neither temp will properly bake the cake. Now envision yourself at the registration desk of an emergency department, trying to check patients in with a nonfunctioning computer, or as a nurse on a hospital floor trying to distribute medicines without access to the patient records, or as a surgeon unsure whether they can start a case out of fear that the anesthesia monitoring equipment is failing to connect to the hospital network, which may affect safeguards.

During the e-mail exchange with the *BMJ* editor, they asked me if there was anything that we could do to help the current situation. All that was really possible at that point was to help via education by giving the employees, families, and patients at NHS information that would help them better understand but that also might assist in preventing the attack from spreading or worsening. Several days later, we published a piece in an effort to help educate and prevent spread of the attack. The approach of the piece, modeling cybersecurity as infection prevention and control is something that occurred to me several years earlier while working on Ebola relief efforts in Sierra Leone. The concept was simple: Take a set of highly familiar concepts and processes and present cybersecurity responses to the "infection" of a cyberattack based upon the NHS clinical guidance for Healthcare Associated Infections: Prevention and Control in Primary and Community Care.[20] I received feedback almost immediately telling me how helpful this model was and that it is still used and referred to by healthcare workers.

Because the impacts were so far reaching, the WannaCry cyberattack did serve as a cyber wake-up call to many industries around the world. The global cost estimate approaches $4 billion and the effects were felt far beyond health care and the NHS.[21] These estimates are difficult to confirm for many reasons, not the least of which is that WannaCry was followed a month later by a highly destructive variant referred to as Petya. This variant was not ransomware, but a wiper disguised as ransomware that was even more destructive.[22]

According to Interpol and the BBC, just 72 hours after being discovered the WannaCry attack had reached 200,000 computers in more than 150 countries.[23] Victims included: The Interior Ministry of Russia; German railways; Chinese universities; the state police in India; Spanish telecoms; Federal Express in the United States; and small and medium-sized businesses in Australia. The attack was quick, silent, and worldwide within hours in a manner that had never been experienced. In many ways, the world awoke to a science fiction novel that weekend, and, we can hope, learned lessons that will make us all safer in the long-term.

One of the more interesting stories from WannaCry was that of Marcus Hutchins, then a 22-year-old a cybersecurity researcher who has been credited with finding and communicating a "kill switch" that slowed the outbreak and then for fighting the worm that crippled Britain's hospital network as well as factories, government agencies, banks, and other businesses around the world.[24] According to NBC News, "Hutchins said he stumbled across the solution when he was analyzing a sample of the malicious code and noticed it was linked to an unregistered web address. He promptly registered the domain, something he regularly does to discover ways to track or stop cyber threats and found that stopped the worm from spreading." This information then enabled others to do likewise. As we discussed earlier, the "lone hacker" paradigm, the fact that an enabled individual can wage asymmetrical war against a far larger and more powerful adversary, was once again proven to be accurate; although this time, the hacker was wearing a white hat instead of black. Interestingly, hackers may have hats of multiple colors, because Hutchins was arrested just a few months later in Las Vegas, Nevada by federal marshals who alleged that he developed Kronos, a malware that steals banking credentials from the browsers of infected computers. The indictment also accused him of developing another malware known as the UPAS Kit. Hutchins was released on a $30,000 bond.[25] The charges were based upon crimes committed in his youth, long before his heroics earlier that year. He was eventually sentenced to supervised release and did not do jail time.

Other than well-documented outages, appointment cancellations, and longer wait times, the complete effects of the WannaCry attack on the NHS and other healthcare facilities remains somewhat unknown. This is not for lack of effort but because health care is very, very good at counting and measuring certain things, such as procedures, and very, very poor at measuring other things, such as whether a patient seen regularly at a hospital has died. Some of this was discussed in the chapters on electronic medical records, because some believe that greater technological interoperability among healthcare computer systems will solve the issues. I see this a bit differently. Yes, better interoperability will help. Of course, it will, but it is not a fix for limited questions or when people are not asking the right questions. For example, it is easy to measure statistics around emergency room appointments/visits on the day of a cyberattack and compare them with historical records for the same day in other years, other days that week, other days that month, etc., and this has all been done. What is far more difficult is predicting the impact of events that haven't happened or happened at a different place. For example, a patient hears that a NHS hospital is closed due to a cyberattack, so they decide not to seek care for what might be a serious situation. Alternatively, a patient cancels an appointment for a cancer screening and doesn't get around to rescheduling. There are almost infinite permutations of this, and many would not be "countable" within single institutions let alone across institutions. According to a WannaCry Impact piece in the journal *Nature*,

It is difficult to capture the true impact of the cyberattack, as mortality is a crude measure of patient harm and there is no current way to quantify patient harm, lapses, and patient safety. If computer systems were down, staff would also be unable to report any patient safety incidents that would otherwise be reported using the NRLS. This is also true for the recording of any data/events during the WannaCry period.[26]

Eventually, it was determined that North Korea was behind the WannaCry attacks. The announcement came in the form of an opinion-editorial in *The Wall Street Journal* authored by President Donald Trump's Homeland Security Advisor, Thomas Bossert.[27] "We do not make this allegation lightly. It is based on evidence. We are not alone with our findings, either. Other governments and private companies agree . . . ," Bossert writes. "The consequences and repercussions of WannaCry were beyond economic. The malicious software hit computers in the UK's health-care sector particularly hard, compromising systems that perform critical work. These disruptions put lives at risk."

It is interesting to think a bit more deeply about what happened here. We often talk about cyberwarfare as though it is science fiction or some background game of chess being waged behind closed doorways deep within governments. The truth is that it is being waged in the open and, often, without consequence. In a shooting war, the bloodshed is all too real and understandable, but in cyberwar the victims may never even know they are casualties. A stark example of this would be to compare WannaCry theoretically to a physical situation wherein North Korean troops landed on UK soil and blockaded hospitals, separating UK citizens from essential care. What would be the government response to that? When the UK made public their findings that North Korea was behind the attack, according to BBC *Today*,

[T]he security minister Ben Wallace said the government now believes a North Korean hacking group was responsible but stopped short of suggesting the UK could carry out retaliatory attacks.[28] [Further], Asked what the UK could do in response to the attack, the minister admitted that it would be "challenging" to arrest anyone when a "hostile state" was involved. He called on the West to instead develop a "doctrine of deterrent" similar to that used to prevent the use of nuclear weapons. "We do have a counterattack capability," he said. "But let's remember we are an open liberal democracy with a large reliance on IT systems. We will obviously have a different risk appetite. If you get into 'tit for tat' there has to be serious consideration of the risks, we would expose UK citizens to.

In my opinion, this question requires a great deal of thought by national and healthcare security experts worldwide. In truth, heavily sanctioned nation states such as North Korea actually have very little to fear short of a shooting war; and effective deterrents are truly needed.

Lessons learned and not learned

So, what did we learn from WannaCry? In my opinion, the number one lesson that should have been learned is that cybervulnerability is not as directly linked to the strength of the components of solid cybersecurity programs as might be thought at first glance. Said differently, good cyberpractices will not protect poor information technology (IT) practices. The organizations most affected by WannaCry were first and foremost NOT practicing solid IT fundamentals. They were behind on systems patching or the systems were unpatched altogether. Many affected machines were running very old versions of operating systems, which were embedded within complex systems and this wasn't always known or recognized.[29] From a technology perspective, building a strong fence around a house that is crumbling is unlikely to keep the house from falling down. It only takes a little wind. Second, with respect to cyberpreparedness, the gaps were the most typical ones. Untested backup strategies failed. There were no clear chains of command, incident-response capabilities failed, and those in authority did not anticipate how their own defensive moves would hinder their own responses. In other words, lots of stuff going wrong and poor preparation was the cause of most of it.

This interplay and interdependency between solid technology management fundamentals and credible cybersecurity management, testing, and oversight is what I feel may not have been understood and learned. Certainly not as clearly as it should have been. Some organizations were not affected because they were prepared. We can hope they stay that way. Some organizations have improved basic management practices, and some have improved their cybercapabilities. It is unclear how many have improved both. To my eye, when visiting and consulting at facilities, I feel that most are trying but still do not really "get it" the way they should. Let's hope that it does not take another WannaCry to truly drive these points home.

The case studies presented here were selected for their impact and notoriety, and as examples of principles, or the lack of the application of principles, within this book. New attacks are occurring daily and to the individual victims the impacts range from annoying to devastating. Health care has begun to put in the requisite effort, investment, and prioritization, but it is still not even close to fully understanding or mitigating cyberthreats to patient safety.

References

1. Strickland E. 5 Major Hospital Hacks: Horror Stories from the Cybersecurity Front Lines. *IEEE Spectrum*. 2016, March 15.
2. Allen J. Terrorizing Civilians and Bombing Hospitals Is a Core Part of Assad's Strategy. CNN. 2019, September 2.
3. Lemos R. Attacks on Healthcare Jump 60% in 2019—So Far. *Dark Reading*. 2019, November 14. Accessed December 2019. https://www.darkreading.com/threat-intelligence/attacks-on-healthcare-jump-60--in-2019---so-far/d/d-id/1336364
4. Albanesius C. Target and the 10 Biggest Hacks of 2013. *PC Magazine*. 2013, December 19.
5. Nigrin DJ. When "Hacktivists" Target Your Hospital. *New England Journal of Medicine* 2014. 371(5):393–395. doi:10.1056/NEJMp1407326
6. Trend Micro. Hacktivism 101: A Brief History and Timeline of Notable Events. 2015, August 17. Accessed November 2019. https://www.trendmicro.com/vinfo/us/security/news/cyber-attacks/hacktivism-101-a-brief-history-of-notable-incidents
7. Dietsche E. Boston Children's Hospital Hacker Sentenced to 10 Years in Prison. *MedCityNews*. 2019, January 14. Accessed December 2019. https://medcitynews.com/2019/01/boston-childrens-hospital-hacker/?rf=1
8. Perakslis ED. Cybersecurity in Health Care. *New England Journal of Medicine* 2014. 371(5):395–397. doi:10.1056/NEJMp1404358
9. Palozza F. The Origin of Ransomware and Its Impact on Businesses. *Radware Blog*. 2018, October 4.
10. Federal Bureau of Investigation. Incidents of Ransomware on the Rise. Protect Yourself and Your Organization. 2016, April 29. Accessed December 2019. https://www.fbi.gov/news/stories/incidents-of-ransomware-on-the-rise
11. American Medical Association. Patient Safety: The Importance of Cybersecurity in Healthcare. 2018. Accessed December 2019. https://www.ama-assn.org/system/files/2018-10/cybersecurity-health-care-infographic.pdf
12. Robeznieks A. Cybersecurity: Ransomware Attacks Shut Down Clinics, Hospitals. American Medical Association. 2019, October 4. Accessed December 2019. https://www.ama-assn.org/practice-management/sustainability/cybersecurity-ransomware-attacks-shut-down-clinics-hospitals
13. Garrity M. 15 Notable Ransomware Attacks on Healthcare Providers in 2019. *Becker's Hospital Report*. 2019, December 18.
14. United Kingdom National Audit Office. Investigation: WannaCry Cyber Attack and the NHS. 2018, April. HC 414 SESSION 2017–2019 25
15. Ghafur S, S Kristensen, K Honeyford, G Martin, A Darzi, and P Aylin. A Retrospective Impact Analysis of the WannaCry Cyberattack on the NHS. *NPJ Digital Medicine* 2019. 2:98. doi:10.1038/s41746-019-0161-6
16. Krebs on Security. Study: Ransomware, Data Breaches at Hospitals Tied to Uptick in Heart Attacks. 2019, November 7. Accessed December 2019. https://krebsonsecurity.com/tag/wannacry/
17. Choi SJ, ME Johnson, and CU Lehmann. Data Breach Remediation Efforts and Their Implications for Hospital Quality. *Health Services Research* 2019. 54(5):971–980. doi:10.1111/1475-6773.13203

18. Spitzer J. Hospitals Aren't Buying Cybersecurity Insurance, FICO Survey Finds. *Becker's Hospital Review*. 2018, August 22.

19. Hayden ME. A Timeline of the WannaCry Cyberattack. ABC News. 2017, May 15.

20. National Institute for Health and Care Excellence. Healthcare-Associated Infections: Prevention and Control in Primary and Community Care. *Clinical Guideline CG139*. 2017, February.

21. Berr J. WannaCry Ransomware Attack Losses Could Reach $4.0 Billion. CBS News. 2017, May 16.

22. Quora. How Similar Are WannaCry and Petya Ransomware? *Forbes*. 2017, July 5.

23. BBC News. Ransomware Cyber-Attack: Who Has Been Hardest Hit? BBC. 2017, May 15.

24. Associated Press. Marcus Hutchins "Saved the US" from WannaCry Cyberattack on Bedroom Computer. NBC News. 2017, May 16.

25. Whittaker Z. Marcus Hutchins, Malware Researcher and "WannaCry Hero," Sentenced to Supervised Release. TechCrunch. 2019, July 26.

26. Ghafur S, S Kristensen, K Honeyford, G Martin, A Darzi, and P Aylin. A Retrospective Impact Analysis of the WannaCry Cyberattack on the NHS. *NPJ Digital Medicine* 2019. 2:98.

27. Stat N. US Declares North Korea the Culprit Behind Devastating WannaCry Ransomware Attack. *The Verge*. 2017, December 18.

28. Withnall A. British Security Minister Says North Korea Was Behind WannaCry Hack on NHS. *The Independent*. 2017, October 27.

29. Bristol CM. Ten Lessons from the Report on the NHS WannaCry Cyberattack. BC Training. 2017, November 3. Accessed December 2019. https://www.b-c-training.com/bulletin/10-lessons-from-the-report-on-the-nhs-wannacry-cyber-attack

PART 4

DIGITAL HEALTH—HOPE, HYPE, AND RISK MITIGATION IN PRACTICE

16
The "Smart" Clinic

A "smart" device is an electronic device, generally connected to other devices or networks via various wireless protocols, such as Bluetooth or Wi-Fi that can operate to some extent interactively and autonomously.[1] The term also is often associated with the concept of ubiquitous computing, the idea that computing can happen anywhere or anytime as opposed to computing that is locked to a desktop computer. Originating in the 1960s, smart devices entered the consumer market in the late 1990s but did not achieve widespread use until the early to mid-2010s. A 2012 consumer report that pulled data from the National Association of Home Builders looked at what kinds of smart-home devices homeowners wanted most and found that the top five were wireless security systems (50%), programmable thermostats (47%), security cameras (40%), lighting control systems (39%), wireless home audio systems (39%), home theater systems (37%), and multizone HVAC systems (37%).[2]

Just as quickly as smart devices entered the consumer market, they became targets for cyberattack. On October 21, 2016, a massive DDOS attack caused widespread disruption of the Internet. Everything from online shopping, to social media and core business activities at some companies were disrupted and offline for hours or longer. The nature of the attacks was the direction of huge amounts of bogus traffic at targeted servers, namely those belonging to Dyn, a company that is a major provider of DNS services to other companies.[3] Major websites were affected, including Twitter, Pinterest, Reddit, GitHub, Etsy, Tumblr, Spotify, PayPal, Verizon, Comcast, and the Playstation network. The attacks were facilitated by the large number of unsecured Internet-connected digital devices, such as home routers and surveillance cameras that used default passwords. Because the default passwords for most devices are widely known, anyone placing such a device on the Internet without first changing the default password is, in effect, facilitating attacks of this type. According to a blogpost a few days after the attack from Morey Haber, Chief Technology and Chief Information Security Officer at the cybersecurity firm BeyondTrust, "Sure, thieves, criminals, and malicious entities will always exist, but IoT [Internet of Things] devices are the dumbest and simplest devices connected to the Internet." This demonstrates the paradox that

Digital Health. Eric D. Perakslis and Martin Stanley, Oxford University Press (2021). © Oxford University Press.
DOI: 10.1093/oso/9780197503133.003.0016

"smart" devices are often "dumb" with respect to privacy and security. That said, consumer technology will never be frozen in time. The nature of technology is advancement, especially where there is clear unmet need, such as in the case of human health and medicine.

Despite the risks and harsh realities, investment in smart technologies in most sectors continues to grow. Smart-city investments include smart utility meters, traffic signals, Wi-Fi kiosks, e-governance applications, and even radio-frequency identification (RFID) sensors within pavement.[5] All of this is based upon the hope that the resulting data will make everything from financial management to bus scheduling more efficient.[6] Smart banking is already changing consumer experiences via banker mobility, next-generation self-service, remote advisory, social computing, and the use of digital signage, all in the hope that technologies such as blockchain and artificial intelligence will optimize it all on the back end.[7] Although some of these approaches offer incremental or questionable benefits, others are clearly bringing significant value. For example, the construction industry remains one of the most dangerous with the U.S. Census Bureau reporting 937 fatalities in 2015. Using drones and other digital technologies, crews can reduce human participation in dangerous inspections and other tasks, which could ensure that the human workers are entering a site only when it is safe to do so, reducing the likelihood of accidents.[8] From automated sensors and autonomous farm vehicles to almost human-free manufacturing facilities, few areas of endeavor are free from this march of technology.

As one of the most complex ecosystems, health care is testing many of these advancements, leading to change from both without and within. Although none of these changes are inherently bad, what must be understood is the sum total of the risk as it is compounded. I discussed the early effects of this additive exposure in a *BMJ* blog post in January 2018.[9] All too often, the default Internet connectivity setting is "on," which is the root of the problem. For example, connecting an implantable pacemaker to the Internet allows for software updates to be automated, the device's performance to be monitored, and even the patient's physiology to be tracked. This functionality confers clear benefits to the device manufacturer from the standpoint of quality control and risk management. It also offers potential benefits for patients, but what are the corresponding risks? Could hackers disrupt the device? Could loss of signal lead to a perception of device malfunction, possibly leading to unnecessary procedures? What about patient privacy? These types of attacks are clearly possible, but how do we calculate the medical risk-benefit ratio? Unlike hospital-acquired infections, adverse drug reactions, and other well-quantified models of medical risk-benefit, we have no clear or common frameworks for cyberthreats in health care. Yet, with U.S. hospitals currently having on average 10 to 15 connected devices per bed, we desperately need them.

Interestingly, although calculating the risk-benefit ratio of implantable pacemakers and other medical devices is complex, we are increasingly encountering another kind of situation wherein the tradeoffs are clear. More and more, we are bombarded with marketing and pop science content promoting gadgets, appliances, and devices with Internet connectivity. Even if they are not medical devices, and serve no purpose in the care of patients, these appliances and gadgets can potentially compromise healthcare systems simply by being part of the patient-care environment. Using the infection-control metaphor of my previous *BMJ* Opinion piece, connected devices are infection vectors and their chains of transmission can be complex.[10] For example, consider a grade-school child who connects their laptop or phone to the wireless network at their school and at home. Now assume that the child has a parent who connects their phone to that same home network, as well as to the hospital network where they are employed. You now have a viable chain of transmission from a public elementary school to a hospital network. Not only is this chain of access viable, it is actually attractive, given that the hackers can target any institution indirectly, which provides a layer of misdirection that can shield their actions from investigation. This happens every day.

Where are the lists and/or warning labels containing the essential benefits to offset the cyberrisks of IoT devices and appliances? How "wired" should even the most modern hospitals be? Healthcare workers, administrators, and engineers have the opportunity to exert control over cyberthreats within their environments by simply keeping these things in mind when managing the physical clinical environment. The simple truth is that cyberrisk decreases as the number of connected devices (endpoints) and the complexity of the environment is decreased. Are the net benefits of these technologies clear and adequate enough to offset the associated risks?

Realizing the promise of smart devices in the clinic today and tomorrow

As previously discussed, with the exception of electronic health records (EHRs), few major technical changes have occurred in most modalities of clinical care, but some of the visions are compelling and some innovations appear closer to realization than others. Of course, these visions are highly dependent upon whom you ask. Technology companies paint one version, clinicians and hospital administrators paint another. Of course, it may be best to start with a patient perspective. In an excellent blogpost in May 2018, Dr. Anees Fareed shared his wife's thoughts on the topic,

> Once I check in to a hospital, the whole journey should be seamless without the long queues at multiple counters for various administrative purposes or clinical tests, all these should be just that click away. I would never ever be burdened with that hefty folder of tests and results, all information required for my treatment should be readily available to all care providers, and finally when I return back home I should have access to relevant information to continue my treatment and stay healthy, such a hospital," she exclaimed, "would indeed be smart.[11]

Said differently, her answer described a better patient experience, improved efficiency of patient services and care processes that ensures seamless patient flow and access to relevant information for both healthcare providers and patients. Well said.

But how to get to that better patient experience? Interestingly, there are many similarities among the things that register as important in surveys on clinical care and clinical research. First, such wish lists often start with mundane and often nonmedical elements, such as parking or more easily navigated public transportation.[12] Similarly, requests for less convoluted appointment scheduling and reminder systems, easier to understand forms, shorter wait times, cleaner and more comfortable waiting areas, and better online communication tend to rise to the top of these types of lists.[13] Clearly, digital tools are ideally suited to deliver on these opportunities. From better e-mail and SMS-text scheduling and reminders, to simple parking apps and telehealth, many advancements in smart cities and towns should be readily adaptable by healthcare institutions that can afford to do so. Another important set of opportunities for improved patient experience lie in quality and safety. As previously discussed, healthcare delivery settings are, unfortunately, far more hazardous to patients than they should be. Using technologies to ensure better real-time communication with patients to prevent slips and falls, to analyze situations, and to flag high-risk patients, staff, and situations for potential accidents should be high on any hospital's lists.

Along these lines, the Agency for Healthcare Research and Quality (AHRQ) administers a program called the Consumer Assessment of Healthcare Providers and Systems (CAHPS). The purpose of the program is to advance the scientific understanding of the patient experience with healthcare.[14] In use since 1995, CAHPS data incentivizes focus on patient experience through the use of scores for quality-based reimbursement on the state and federal levels, as well as through the public release of scoring information that incentivizes recognition and action by health systems. According to AHRQ, CAPHS data reinforce opportunities for better patient experience to improve clinical care, to reduce risks, and to improve business profitability. For example, improved patient experiences correlate with better adherence to medical advice and treatment plans, better outcomes, lower malpractice risk, and better employee satisfaction and retention, as well as relationship quality and retention.

Another interesting trend (and debate) is that patient experiences can be improved by treating patients more like retail customers. There is a bit of inevitability to this. As copays increase for many patients, comparison shopping is inevitable. Advocates for the approach argue for a shift in power dynamics from an authoritarian doctor-as-commander interaction to an empowered consumer role that gives patients more control and responsibility.[15] It is hoped that this shift will improve communication, make patients more directly active and engaged, and help build better trust and loyalty. Take the element of decision-making, for example; do we really know how many patients feel as in charge of important healthcare decisions as they feel when selecting a new car? Do they spend as much time shopping? Do they ask around for references? Do they utilize as many sources of data? All of these are interesting questions and the school of thought that advocates for more consumerism in health care is actively running the experiments now.[16]

Conversely, some feel that patients are not customers and should not be treated as such. Shirie Leng, MD describes this viewpoint,

> Patients are not on vacation. They are not in the mindset that they are sitting in the doctor's office or the hospital to have a good time. They are not relaxed. They have not left their troubles temporarily behind them. They have not bought room service and a massage. They are not in the mood to be happy. They would rather not be requiring the service they are requesting. Which leads to number 2, Patients have not chosen to buy the service. Patients have been forced to seek the service, in most cases. Patients are not paying for the service . . . and they have no idea what the price is anyway . . . .[17]

Clearly these are compelling statements and must be kept in mind as design input.

Another element to consider is the explosive growth of direct-to-consumer "health" products. Contrary to Dr Leng's second point in the previous section, many patients are actually choosing to consume optional "healthcare" services. The consumer genomics market is a good example. It is estimated that more than 30 million people have opted to participate in the consumer genomics market with 23andMe having sold approximately 10 million tests at the time of this writing.[18] These are impressive numbers to be sure; although the sales appear to have plateaued and are now on the decline. Reasons for the decline appear to be privacy concerns and ambiguity regarding validity and usefulness of the data. In short, patients appear to be learning that "medical" data that poses more questions than it answers, is of little possible value and may even be a net negative experience.

Looking at the digital clinic of the future, many predict that it is all about experience and potentially high-end experiences at that. A *Business Insider* piece from 2018 on Lab100, a joint venture between the research institute at Mount Sinai and Cactus Design Studio sported the headline, "Mount Sinai teamed up with the designers who created projects for Nike and Beyonce to build a futuristic, new clinic—and it's reimagining how healthcare is delivered."[19] Hype aside, Lab100 seeks to provide digital solutions to some of the more practical challenges in health care today. For example, there is a significant focus on wellness and prevention, concerns that are frequently cited as priorities for healthcare systems but seldom brought to fruition, given that most healthcare providers are simply too busy caring for the sick and injured. Wellness has been considered an ideal use for digital health since the beginning. Pedometers, GPS-enabled watches, smartwatches, Fitbit-like activity trackers, and health-focused mobile apps have been used by hundreds of millions of consumers world-wide. This has created ambiguous spaces around fitness, health, and wellness, as well as between the consumer electronics industry and traditional medical equipment manufacturers.

For now, it is important to note that the basic premise of many visions for the smart clinic of the future is experiential versus substantial. One view is that healthcare delivery will stay mostly the same or change incrementally as more smart devices are put into use by patients themselves or by clinicians and their healthcare institutions. This vision is difficult to debate, given that it describes the world of today quite well, and it assumes that change will continue to happen essentially in the same way that it has already happened, that is, incrementally. At the other end of the scale is a much grander vision, which is based upon technology and data-enabled change that genuinely changes the workflow and basics of healthcare delivery. For example, could smart identification make the registration office at the entrance to clinics as unnecessary as human-operated toll booths on highways that have already been replaced by what are essentially the exact same technologies: RFID tags and smart readers? Would smart operating rooms immediately notify clinical personnel if a patient was in the wrong place and, potentially, receiving the wrong diagnostic test or interventional procedure? One must admit that it is fascinating that relatively simple technologies, applied to the most mundane problems, can often lead to the greatest gains. Then, inevitably, if such good can come from solving "simpler" problems, how great might the rewards be for solving far more complex challenges?

It is difficult to be skeptical in the face of such opportunities, especially when most of the technologies are already available and well-proven. With technical feasibility within reach, the questions should then turn to solid benefit-risk analysis. What are the privacy, security and safety implications of such processes and systems? And what are the potential errors and harms?

References

1. Wikipedia. Smart Device. Accessed November 2019. https://en.wikipedia.org/wiki/Smart_device
2. National Association of Home Builders. "What Homeowners Want." *Home Tech Integration*. Retrieved from Wikipedia. 2019, November 7.
3. Cobb S. 10 Things to Know About the October 21 IoT DDOS Attacks. WeLiveSecurity. 2016, October 24. Accessed November 2019. https://www.welivesecurity.com/2016/10/24/10-things-know-october-21-iot-ddos-attacks/
4. Beyond Trust. IoT Bots Cause Massive Internet Outage October 21, 2016. 2016, October 24. Accessed November 2019. https://www.beyondtrust.com/blog/entry/iot-bots-cause-october-21st-2016-massive-internet-outage
5. Maddox T. 66% of US cities are investing in smart city technology. *Tech Republic*. 2017, November 6.
6. Demos T. "Smart" Technology Could Change the Future of City Finances. *Wall Street Journal*. 2019, June 10.
7. Stokes A. Introducing Smart Banking: The Future of Banking. TheRecord. 2014, May 22. Accessed November 2019. https://www.technologyrecord.com/Article/introducing-smart-banking-the-future-of-banking-26700
8. Zinkel B. The Rise of Smart Technology Within The Construction Industry. Transportation Safety Apparel. 2017, December 26. https://www.procore.com/jobsite/smart-apparel-the-future-of-wearable-technology-on-the-jobsite/. Accessed December 2019.
9. Perakslis E. It's Time to Address the Medical Benefits and Risks of the Internet of Things. *BMJ Blog*. 2018, January 29.
10. Perakslis E. Cyber Security Modeled as Infection Prevention and Control in the Healthcare Delivery Setting. *BMJ Blog*. 2017, May 16. https://blogs.bmj.com/bmj/2018/01/29/eric-d-perakslis-its-time-to-address-the-medical-benefits-and-risks-of-the-internet-of-things/
11. Fareed A. Building Strategy for Smart Hospitals. *Cerner Blog*. 2018, May 22. Accessed December 2019. https://www.cerner.com/ae/en/blog/building-strategy-for-smart-hospitals
12. Ziv S. How to Design a Better Clinical Trial with the Patient Experience in Mind. *Newsweek*. 2017, July 21.
13. PatientPop.com. 12 Actionable Ideas to Improve Patient Experience. 2019, April 23. Accessed December 2019. https://www.patientpop.com/blog/running-a-practice/patient-experience/ideas-to-improve-patient-experience/

14. AHRQ. About CAHPS. 2020, January. Accessed January 2020. https://www.ahr q.gov/cahps/about-cahps/index.html

15. Stamp B. How Thinking of Patients as Customers Can Improve Healthcare. *Becker's Hospital Review*. 2018, October 23.

16. Gingiss D. Why Treating Patients as Consumers Can Improve the Healthcare Experience. *Forbes*. 2019, July 9.

17. Leng S. Patients are NOT Consumers. *The Health Care Blog*. 2015, March 21. https://thehealthcareblog.com/blog/2015/03/21/patients-are-not-customers/

18. Farr C. Consumer DNA Testing Has Hit a Lull—Here's How It Could Capture the Next Wave of Users. CNBC. 2019, August 25.

19. Hu C. Mount Sinai Teamed Up with the Designers Who Created Projects for Nike and Beyonce to Build a Futuristic, New Clinic—And It's Reimagining How Healthcare Is Delivered. *Business Insider*. 2018, August 10.

17

The Patient as a Mobile Health Care Consumer

In the last chapter, we introduced the links and overlaps among health care, health, and wellness within the domain of wearable technologies. For many people, these merge in ways that are not yet easily understood from the standpoint of effectiveness and utility, something I learned firsthand during my own cancer journey. In January of 2005, I had just been promoted to Vice President at Johnson & Johnson. My wife and I were enjoying the absolute chaos that the gift of our 30-month old daughter had brought to our lives, and we had just completed an initial set of renovations on our new home. Things could not have been better when I was diagnosed with advanced renal cancer at the age of 38. Cancer was already a significant shadow in our lives. My father had passed away in 1986 at the age of 42 from head and neck cancer, and two years earlier, I watched a close cousin and his 17-year old daughter both die of cancer within a year of each other. We were clearly sensitized, and my diagnosis landed directly upon this barely managed concern.

I underwent an open partial nephrectomy to remove the cancerous tissue and was placed on active surveillance. This was several years before the progress made by tyrosine kinase inhibitors, so there were no targeted therapies available. Further, my pathology confirmed a papillary subtype, which is less common, representing only about 10% of renal cell carcinoma (RCC) diagnosis. As I recovered on the sofa from my surgery, I watched my daughter rage about the house as only a toddler can do. Being a data science guy, I had done the math. At that time, the statistics suggested that I had roughly a 30% chance of five-year survival. For about a week, all I could think about was that I had roughly a one-in-three chance of seeing that little girl finish third grade. Crazy, I know, but really hard to avoid. Fortunately, the body heals quickly and that healing also soothes the mind. By the time I was off the couch and moving around, I had forcibly expelled those thoughts from my mind, but I also knew I needed to replace them with something. There was no treatment available. No pill I could take. Nothing to be injected into my arm. Nothing active I could do but wait six months and see what the CAT scan showed.

Digital Health. Eric D. Perakslis and Martin Stanley, Oxford University Press (2021). © Oxford University Press.
DOI: 10.1093/oso/9780197503133.003.0017

Given that health care had nothing active to allow me a sense of feeling in control, I switched my focus to wellness.

I started moving to give myself something to do but also for pain control. For whatever reason, I have always had a sensitivity to narcotic pain killers. They give me severe migraine headaches, so I had few options for pain control other than simply moving my body. First, I just walked around the yard. One hand holding the fluid drain from my kidney, the other used for balance and stability. As winter wore on, I felt imprisoned by the weather until I purchased a treadmill that enabled exercise with fewer potential hazards. The treadmill not only enabled safe exercise 24-hours per day on demand, it also displayed data! With precise timing, I could extend my walks by a minute or two each session. Each increase in time and distance felt like progress and transformed passive data into mental and physical goals. As those goals progressed, my energy, strength, and feeling of wellness also progressed. Cancer lost mind-space to endorphins—and not just for me. My wife, Lisa Gail, had lived through most of my family cancer trauma. She seldom spoke of it, but, I assume, she was quietly terrified until she saw my physical appearance, energy, mood, and vigor improving so visibly. Walking became running as winter turned to spring, and Lisa Gail presented me with my first running watch so I could track my progress. I was hooked. I started biking and worked my way up to hundred-mile weeks. My running progressed and a year after my surgery, I completed my first half marathon. A year after that, I completed my first marathon. I became an active patient advocate and even made the cover of *CR Magazine* published by the American Association of Cancer Research (AACR).

To quickly wrap up my story, I remained cancer free for eight years before an annual scan detected recurrence. The recurrence was quickly treated with new less-invasive tools, cryotherapy in my case, and I remain on active surveillance, but without mortal fear. I am living proof that once-deadly diseases can be managed as chronic but non-life-threatening conditions, and I am immensely thankful. That said, truth be told, I have no idea if my focus on wellness and activity is in any way responsible for my happy outcome. Most of the science is yet to be studied, given the complexities of disease, wellness, placebo effect, and many other potential mitigating variables.

During this same period of time activity tracking grew from being an athlete-only pursuit to becoming a more mainstream activity, chiefly via low-cost consumer devices such as FitBit.[1] There are many other players, large and small, in the mix, and they are all selling fitness, wellness, and health as if the concepts were synonymous and well understood. A relatively harmless over-sight in this space, given that almost universally, increased activity is thought to be healthy. Add an electrocardiogram to that same activity tracker, how-ever, and the benefit-risk equation changes rapidly, as we will discuss later.

Telehealth and remote care

Another solid, well-understood, and more direct example is telehealth, which has recently emerged as an essential tool against COVID-19. Broadly de-fined as the remote provision of health care by means of telecommunications technology, the telehealth field continues to grow rapidly. According to the American Medical Association, telehealth is the fastest growing segment of care delivery, increasing in incidence 53% between 2016 and 2017.[2] Telehealth provides the opportunity to bring both basic and highly specialized care to re-mote areas. Although many of the drivers are financial in nature, telehealth also brings significant convenience. According to InTouch Health, telehealth platforms bring, "automatic appointment reminders, stress-free in-app sched-uling tools, and remote physician consultations . . . .Patients no longer have to cross physical barriers to speak with a healthcare provider, changing the way the average person interacts with the healthcare system."[3]

The opportunities and convenience here are obvious and real. Check-in often is automated through apps that already have the patient identification and insurance information. The wait time effectively goes to zero because the patient can remain engaged in ongoing activities until the visit starts. If labs, imaging, or other tests are required, the patient need only visit those locations. Facilities and all associated expenses can be reduced, as can office and clerical staff. Estimates for actual cost savings range from $19 to $120 per office visit and up to $1,500 per visit when highly expensive visits to hospital emergency rooms can be avoided via diversion to lower-cost care options based upon risk and need.[4]

Of course, nothing is a panacea in health care, and telehealth faces the same scrutiny as all emerging technologies. Starting with the basic premise, there are many clinical interactions where much more than conversation and visual inspection are required. Consults that require detailed physical exam-ination and data collection by even simple instruments that are not yet ubiq-uitous as digital tools, such as blood pressure cuffs and body weight scales, still necessitate physical visits. There is also the issue of trust and privacy. Clinical interactions are traditionally intimate, and many on both sides of the telehealth screen may struggle to feel connected with each other during remote and virtual interactions.[5] In addition, there can be genuine fear of misdiagnosis or other errors. In telemedicine, clinicians are frequently asked to provide care similar to an office visit but with much less data. Studies are mixed and potentially dependent on the health discipline. One study of telemedicine use in skin diseases reported significant misdiagnosis, while another study showed no difference in mortality in patients receiving telehealth care for heart failure.[6,7]

Further, although telehealth clearly has the potential to lower health costs, some payers are concerned that the convenience of telehealth will lead to overuse and actually drive up healthcare costs. This despite the fact that, as of 2018, 35 states had enacted telehealth parity laws, which mandate that insurers pay for analogous services rendered via telehealth technologies.[8] Economics are complex, and many institutions struggle when trying to understand, realize, and optimize cost savings and cost avoidance opportunities. The long-term effects of telehealth on the financials of healthcare facilities may take years to understand.

The opportunities highlighted here are high-value targets for digital health innovators, starting with the concept of a virtual or remote physical exam. If patients are equipped with adequate biosensor data capture, as well as storage and transmission devices, many hope that the risks of misdiagnosis can be decreased. Instead of a clinician trying to extract as much as possible via conversation and visible observation through a video chat, the interaction can be greatly enhanced if accurate, objective, timely, and bias-free data is available digitally during the interaction. Of course, the accuracy, reliability, and comparability of most remote digital measurement tools is considered experimental at the time of this writing. In addition, the comprehensive benefits and risks of this approach and tools are far from understood.[9]

If we are optimistic, we can expect that parts of traditional health care will be replaced by superior remote options that exceed many of the basic limitations of care today. For example, most "sick" healthcare visits are brief and are capable of only capturing a minute snapshot of diagnostic information or symptoms. Take the difference in the richness of information in a single blood pressure measurement versus a plot of measurements collected at one-minute intervals over the preceding 24 hours. Extrapolate the opportunity for more detailed and time-scaled data across all basic vital signs measurement and the opportunity is far too compelling to ignore, especially when we consider the fact that virtually all adults and many children and adolescents are carrying an Internet-connected digital data collection and transmission device on their person already.

Moving beyond basic healthcare service delivery and into chronic disease management and research, even more new opportunities present. Degenerative neuromuscular diseases, such as multiple sclerosis (MS), can be monitored 24–7–365 via accelerometer-equipped digital phones and watches, which can track symptom progression during every waking and sleeping moment for a given patient. The volume and velocity of this data is not yet digestible in most healthcare settings but is being incorporated into clinical research. At a time when clinical research participation is limited by logistical issues such as time and travel burden on research participants, the ability to virtualize and de-burden the interaction holds great promise for transforming biomedical research and development.[10] Beyond reducing logistical burdens, digital tools can increase the quality of data and feedback participants receive, engage the patient more compellingly through gamification and reward systems for compliance, and increase the odds that the patient will benefit from the trial in more medically meaningful ways. Further, the ability to receive, filter, assess, and utilize real-time streams of data containing millions of observations per patient per day is simply not tractable by the human mind alone—as we will discuss in the next chapter on artificial intelligence. Clearly, decentralizing health care is one of the greatest opportunities for digital health to live up to the hope and hype.

References

1. Fitbit. About Us. Accessed December 2019. https://www.fitbit.com/us/about-us
2. AMA Staff News Writer. Telehealth Up 53%, Growing Faster than Any Other Place of Care. 2019, May 29. Accessed December 2019.https://www.ama-assn.org/practice-management/digital/telehealth-53-growing-faster-any-other-place-care
3. In Touch Health. What's Driving Telehealth Growth in 2019? Accessed December 2019. https://intouchhealth.com/whats-driving-telehealth-growth-in-2019/
4. CheneyC.CostSavingsforTelemedicineEstimatedat$19to$120perVisit.Healthleadersmedia. com. 2019, May 7. Accessed December 2019. https://www.healthleadersmedia.com/clinical-care/cost-savings-telemedicine-estimated-19-120-patient-visit
5. Lipton W. The Problem with Telemedicine. 2018, July 12. Accessed December 2019. https://www.physicianspractice.com/article/problem-telemedicine
6. Beck M. Study of Telemedicine Finds Misdiagnoses of Skin Problems. *Wall Street Journal.* 2016, May 15.
7. Flodgren G et al. Interactive Telemedicine: Effects on Professional Practice and Healthcare Outcomes. 2015, September 7. Accessed December 2019. https://www.cochrane.org/CD002098/EPOC_interactive-telemedicine-effects-professional-practice-and-healthcare-outcomes
8. Restrepo K. The Case Against Telemedicine Parity Laws. John Locke Foundation. 2018, January 15. https://www.johnlocke.org/research/telemedicine/

9. Shieber J. No One Knows How Effective Digital Therapies Are, But a New Tool from Elektra Labs Aims to Change That. *TechCrunch*. 2019, November 12.

10. Fred Hutch Press Release. Research Shows Structural Barriers Are the Biggest Reason for Low Participation in Clinical Trials. 2019, February 19. Accessed December 2019. https://www.fredhutch.org/en/news/releases/2019/02/research-shows-structural-barriers-are-the-biggest-reason-for-low-participation-in-clinical-trials.html

18

Artificial Intelligence in Health Care

A great deal of hype surrounds artificial intelligence (AI) in health care, but what exactly is it? AI can be described as technology that behaves intelligently using skills associated with human intelligence, including the ability to perceive, learn, reason, and act autonomously. Put more simply, AI is a collection of technologies that give machines cognitive capabilities to advise humans and/or carry out their wishes. As aggregated by Dr. Paul Marsden, examples of "working definitions of AI" include: " . . . the science and engineering of making intelligent machines" . . . "[where] intelligence is the computational part of the ability to achieve goals in the world" (original definition by John McCarthy, who coined the term "Artificial Intelligence" in 1955); " . . . the science of making machines do things that would require intelligence if done by men" (definition offered by AI pioneer Marvin Minsky in 1968); " . . . a constellation of technologies that extend human capabilities by sensing, comprehending, acting and learning—allowing people to do much more" (Accenture 's definition).[1] There are many more definitions. None of these are bad or incorrect, but, as the reader might detect, the definitions often are manipulated to target certain markets.

The concepts are exciting for sure but also concerning. According to the Internet Society in a policy brief published in 2017, "As machine learning is used more often in products and services, there are some significant considerations when it comes to users' trust.., including, socio-economic impacts; issues of transparency, bias, and accountability; new uses for data, considerations of security and safety, ethical issues; and, how AI facilitates the creation of new ecosystems."[2] Throughout this chapter, we will be diving into all of these aspects, with a specific focus on healthcare implementations and impacts..

Lastly, with respect to definition, AI is often confused or conflated with similar computing methodologies and capabilities, most notably machine learning. Machine learning (ML) is a subcategory of AI which relies on big data sets to remind the data to find common patterns.[3] The core differences between ML and AI can be described as follows: ML uses the experience to look for the pattern it learned. AI uses the experience to acquire knowledge

Digital Health. Eric D. Perakslis and Martin Stanley, Oxford University Press (2021). © Oxford University Press.
DOI: 10.1093/oso/9780197503133.003.0018

and/or skill and also to learn how to apply that knowledge for new environments. For the sake of this writing, I will not bore the reader by constantly pointing out these differences and specifics. Instead, whenever AI is mentioned, please assume that the application is likely a composite utilization of both technologies as is often the case.

Prevalent current uses

Like most basic computing technologies, AI was first utilized within advanced computing applications and use cases and is now considered a basic technology within this space. The fields of robotics, language and image processing, data mining, and visualization and image recognition are all common applications where AI may be an underlying technology. Cybersecurity applications of AI/ML include monitoring and threat analysis. AI/ML makes sense of the large volume and velocity of data, which is simply impossible for humans to understand, filter, or act upon. ML can seek and define patterns, upon which AI can provide suggestions. According to IBM, "As cyberattacks grow in volume and complexity, artificial intelligence (AI) is helping under-resourced security operations analysts stay ahead of threats . . . , AI provides instant insights to help you fight through the noise of thousands of daily alerts, drastically reducing response times."[5] This marketing text is interesting because it directly speaks to one of the greatest hopes for future uses of AI, namely, human augmentation.

Beyond applications within information technology, AI has steadily and effectively crept into most sectors of the economy. When a check is deposited in a bank via a mobile app that includes a digital image of the check, AI is likely at use analyzing specific attributes of the image, such as the signature. When an online retailer suggests products to a return shopper or a media purveyor such as a news webpage or video streaming service suggests content, the underlying technology is an AI-based recommender system. Although these uses offer convenience, the potential drawbacks must be considered. For example, social media programs have used image analysis on user-posted photos to suggest friends. Convenient? Yes, but also a clear case of video surveillance via the use of personally identifiable data (PII). Another growing use case is personal digital assistants such as Siri from Apple and Alexa for Amazon.[7] These products increase the accessibility of features such as search and text by voice, but unbeknown to the user may also learn private information.

It is these contradictions between utility and privacy, convenience and risk that remain at the heart of debate on the use of AI. Concerns range from the existential risk of losing complete control of our technological world to machines, a la Skynet from the 1980s Terminator movies, to the more subtle and likely threats to privacy and manipulation of facts. All to be discussed later.

As with most emerging technologies, lines form quickly to exploit, debate, and decry the opportunity. At the forefront are technology companies looking to productize the technology. At their side are consulting and service companies looking to capitalize on the integration and implementation opportunities, often in order to quickly replace whatever most recent panacea they had sold. Academics invent, investigate, and debate the pros and cons. In 2019, there were scores of AI-focused conferences or meetings weekly, many boasting more than 200 exhibitors and tens of thousands of attendees.[8] In health care, caution and intellectualism often moderate excitement and many of the technocentric, vendor-driven events are balanced by events such as "*Hype vs. Reality: The Role of AI in Global Health*," held by the Harvard Global Health Institute.[9] At the time of this writing, well-balanced views often are captured by quotes such as this one from Adam Landman, Chief Information Officer at Brigham and Women's Hospital and an associate professor of emergency medicine at Harvard Medical School, "it's important that AI not be viewed as a solution in search of a problem, but that the health care outcomes be considered first and AI considered as one tool among others to address it."

Healthcare use cases for AI are emerging. A literature review of the application of AI and ML in medical image analysis in 2017 identified 58 papers on brain imaging alone, such as machine learning on MRI scans.[10] These use cases included disorder identification, tissue anatomy differentiation, lesion and tumor detection and identification, survival and disease progression prediction, and image enhancement. Similar types of AI/ML image-analysis studies are growing in frequency in retinal image analysis, chest X-rays and CT scans, and other applications in high-content image analysis. Similarly, the field of digital pathology, also a generator of high-content and high-density imaging files is exploding. Because radiology and pathology both traditionally rely on highly trained humans to visually inspect extremely dense and complex images, the opportunity for AI to augment, and possibly replace, these essential skills, represents a clear beachhead for AI in medicine. Indeed, stories such as an *MIT Technology Review* short piece titled, "Google's AI is better at spotting advanced breast cancer than pathologists" that report that an AI/ML tool can detect metastatic cancer 99% of the time, while humans can only do so accurately 38% of the time, are intriguing if not fully convincing.[11] Similar studies in lung cancer, complex pediatric diagnosis, and other multidimensional data-centric medical challenges continue to build the trend.[12,13] As the momentum and the evidence-base grow, the question of whether AI will replace doctors is a subject of growing debate. The likely outcome is that, although AI will not necessarily replace doctors, it is likely to change their jobs and the jobs of other allied health professonals.[14]

Utilization in biomedical research and development

Given the immense costs and the difficult-to-measure efficacy of biomedical research and development (R&D), the search for productivity boosts via new technologies has never been more prolific. Biotechnology companies, as well as biopharmaceutical and medical device companies are sprouting "innovation" groups and hubs in the technology-rich regions of Boston, the Bay Area of northern California, San Francisco, and Asia, all with a competitive eye toward rapid exploitation of the newest technologies. AI intrigues these groups on multiple levels. First, there is the never-ending quest to better understand the complexities of biology. As discussed in the "cures factory" sections, the simple statistical approaches to drug discovery, the idea that machines can design, synthesize, and bioassay large numbers of drug candidate molecules, did not yield the desired fruit. It is enticing to wonder whether trends in these forms of "big data" were missed by the human eye and the numerical methods of the time. Similarly, companies that have spent hundreds of millions of dollars over decades in research and clinical trials, most of which did not succeed, cannot help but wonder whether AI and ML can find the gold in those data that might have been missed. Not only within studies but across studies via data experimentation across data sets or across disease indications. Further, deeper, more revealing, studies of that data may hold insights into basic mechanisms of disease previously unstudied.

The second area of interest and investment concerns leveraging new data into these types of models. The ability to study, and surveil, humans has never been greater. One lab visit can yield tens of thousands of data points via genomics, metabolomics, imaging, and other diagnostic methods. Add in real-time physiological data from wearables and the opportunity to gather information about human health and disease has never been greater. Of course, the ability of humans, or even traditional analytics, to make use of all this data is the challenge of the information age. Take something as simple and traditional and well-understood as heart rate. Easy to measure and easy to interpret, but if heart rate can be measured 15 times per second, 24 hours per day, the result is 86,400 heart rate measurements per day. Is that data still just heart rate or is it a measurement of something else? Apply similar math to dozens or even hundreds of possible physiological measures, and the scientific opportunity is as intriguing as the data management challenge is complex.

The specific effects of the opportunity are currently under study and debate. Although the clear hope is that AI will reduce the cost of predictions, others postulate that it may have an even larger impact on the economy "by serving as a new general-purpose *method of invention* that can reshape the nature of the innovation process and the organization of R&D."[15] The opportunity is not at all limited to the private sector. In June of 2019, the White House released an update to the National Artificial Intelligence Strategic plan originally released in 2016. The plan contains eight strategic priorities: Make long-term investments in AI research; Develop effective methods for human-AI collaboration; Understand and address the ethical, legal, and societal implications of AI; Ensure the safety and security of AI systems; Develop shared public data sets and environments for AI training and testing; Measure and evaluate AI technologies through standards and benchmarks; Better understand the national AI R&D workforce needs; Expand public-private partnerships to accelerate advances in AI.[16] All in all, a comprehensive and solid approach if well executed.

One last area of AI focus within R&D is when the tool itself becomes the product. For example, software as a medical device (SaMD) is defined as software intended to be used for one or more medical purposes that performs these purposes without being part of a hardware medical device.[17] It's an interesting designation because it is difficult to imagine software in the absence of some form of device running the software be it a medical device, cell phone, or wearable, but it is being envisioned and must be considered.

Hazards

Ever since "Hal," the monotone AI character in the movie, *2001: A Space Odyssey*, creeped viewers out in 1968, the concept of malevolent AI has been prime fodder for science fiction. For those fans of the genre, ZNet's rankings of the Top 36 Movies about AI is not to be missed![18] Interestingly, the plots across these movies dating from 1927 are quite apropos. Scenarios range from the "rise of the machines" wherein autonomous computers take over and annihilate humans, to the more subtle situations in which humans are subservient, to the even more subtle situations where humans are unknowingly being manipulated. Some would say, the authors included, that we are, in fact, already living in this latter scenario. Setting aside what is referred to as the existential risk of artificial intelligence, that is, the fear that AI may eventually result in human extinction, there are far more clear and present issues to discuss. There are many ways in which AI is already making our lives better, and there is immense product marketing ever trying to press more of these technologies into all aspects of our lives. The current hazards are also as clear but get far less press or exposure on social media. This quote from Vladimir Putin sums things up well, "Artificial intelligence is the future, not only for Russia, but for all humankind. It comes with enormous opportunities, but also threats that are difficult to predict. Whoever becomes the leader in this sphere will become the ruler of the world.[19]" The battle is already underway in what some refer to as a "warm war." The concept of a warm war exists while both countries are continuing negotiations for a peaceful settlement of tensions but continue to mobilize their forces and implement war plans for an anticipated order to fight.[20] Most national defense professionals would agree that this is our actual current state. It is scary but also inevitable. Every period of modern human history has hosted some form of arms race. For current generations, ours revolves around computers and biology.

Most of us encounter AI in our everyday lives without much recognition. We frequently use recommender systems, personal digital assistants, computer gaming, and even semiautonomous vehicles. The benefits and potential harms of using these narrow AI applications are not always evident. Social manipulation via the targeting of vulnerable groups has been blamed for swaying the outcome of the 2016 presidential election in the United States, and the evidence is quite convincing. Similar tactics are in use in ways that range from simple targeted consumer marketing to social grading, such as is being developed in China with its social credit system that scores people based upon behaviors gleaned from extensive surveillance systems.[21] Very scary and here now.

One significant weakness that has emerged in AL/ML-derived models is that these applications can propagate biases, which can be introduced during training, development, and operation of the AI. If most images of faces in a training set are of Caucasians, the models using this training data will likely struggle to classify faces of other races. The same is true for gender, other physical traits, and even socioeconomic attributes that are collected, aggregated, and modeled in similar fashion. The resulting bias within these programs can lead to significant errors. In one study, the error rates in detecting light-skinned men were on the order of 1%, but the error rate soared to 35% for darker skinned women.[22] This flaw was true even for very high-profile women such as Oprah Winfrey, Michelle Obama, and Serena Williams, which is shocking given that high-profile exemplars most certainly make it into these models. The fear with these issues is further exacerbation of social injustices and widening of economic and social divisions that are already highly problematic worldwide.[23]

The potential hazards of AI in health care are quite broad given the complex relationships between the chances of physical harm, ethical risks and challenges, and legal and socioeconomic hazards. Using the lens of physical harm, medicine must approach the risks from at least four points of view: accidental errors during healthcare provision, malfeasance, charlatanism, and accidental errors by patients and caregivers. Starting with errors in healthcare provision, the most commonly cited concern is with respect to "black box" algorithms. The black box dilemma is based upon the concern that most clinicians do not understand the algorithms being used with AI tools. In fact, AI understandability and explainability are largely open areas of basic AI research and development as noted in the National Artificial Intelligence Research and Development Strategic Plan. Adopters of systems that leverage AI should account and mitigate for the risks associated with the understandability gap by applying metrics or other approaches to avoid the "black box" problem. It is insufficient to use AI systems with just a leap of faith or place trust in something unknown, particularly if a mistake by the AI could cause harm to people. This poses challenges in several ways. The first issue is how to ensure physician trust when AIs model or make recommendations that run counter to historical approaches. Legally, the risk exists that, in a liability setting, clinicians and institutions can be put at risk if trying to justify decisions taken from AI methodologies that they cannot clearly explain in adequate detail.[24] Mitigating this risk will require fundamental changes in medical education but also highly specific approaches to validating AI tools when being implemented in clinical care.[25] Specifically, Andersen and Leigh recommend that "just as medical and ethical expertise should be represented in review board decisions regarding medical practice, so AI expertise should be represented in review board decisions regarding use of AI programs in health care." Clearly this is important but also consequential. Engineering and medicine share many things in common but do not always work so easily together. As we have seen in our study of electronic medical records, the languages of mathematics, engineering, statistics, and medicine do not always comfortably overlap. Practically, there is also the issue that most healthcare delivery institutions, unlike large academic medical centers, do not have ready access to the diverse types of expertise needed to assess these tools and each potential application of them.

Other risks of harm during healthcare provision include accidental misuse, inadequate training, lack of validation or safety checks to catch bias, false positives or false negatives, in the case of diagnostics and improper exploitation for resource management. Considering the latter, in his book, *Deep Medicine: How Artificial Intelligence Can Make Medicine Human Again*, Eric Topol postulates that AI will automate routine tasks and free up time to enable clinicians to spend more time interacting directly with patients.[26] Although we all wish this to be true, the reality of technology utilization in clinical care has been to focus on institutional efficiency as opposed to quality of care. Specifically, time yielded via technological investment has most often been returned to the institution as profit rather than as relaxed expectations of clinician productivity. For example, if an institution works with an AI vendor to automate analysis and interpretation of radiological images, done well, the net value to the institution could be in improved accuracy and reduced human resource requirements. It is possible that the time gains would be passed on to clinicians and enable them to spend more time with each patient, but that would run contrary to the way most relative value units (RVU), the methodology through which most clinicians are compensated, are modeled and determined.[27]

In considering the probabilities and actual risks associated with intentional harms or malfeasance from an adversary, it is first important to understand the concept of attack surface. As described earlier, the attack surface is the summation of inherent risk points within any given system. For any given computer application, the attack surface can be described as the sum of all paths for data/commands into and out of the application, and the code that protects these paths, as well as all valuable data used in the application and the code that protects these data.[28]

So, the more complex, connected, and available any computer application is, the more vulnerable it becomes. Further, in the case of AI, the attack surface includes the algorithms themselves. This can be especially frightening in the case of subtle manipulation, wherein an algorithm is modified just slightly to change results but in a fashion that may be very difficult to detect. Given that most companies in the United States take an average of 206 days to detect a cyberbreach, it is clear that these types of occult attacks can cause a great deal of damage before being discovered; and it can take years to understand the resulting issues.[29] Had the automated services at NHS that were disrupted by the WannaCry automated systems included significant dependency on diagnostic AI, those services also could have gone offline. Further, subtle tampering, such as changing the image of a skin sample to read cancerous versus noncancerous, can be done in ways that are undetectable to the human eye. These types of adversarial attacks are quite complex and sophisticated and must be top priorities for all those who seek to press AI deeply into medical care.[30]

Another important threat to manage is charlatanism. As described earlier, people have been making false claims about medical products for as long as there have been medical products. Charlatanism, misinformation, and disinformation are rampant on the Internet and social media and lead to products and product claims that can be highly coercive and physically harmful.

AI tools on social media are extremely precise and capable of identifying groups who are vulnerable to certain messaging and/or ideology. Today, much of this targeting work is done by human trolls, but, increasingly, the expectation is that these activities will be augmented by AI if not fully automated.[31] Take chatbots as an example. The innocence and helpfulness of Siri and Alexa are quite impressive. Every time a user speaks to an AI assistant, they are teaching it. The assistant knows who the user speaks to, who they text, where they travel and sleep, what restaurants and stores they frequent, and so on. Now imagine subtle manipulation by that same AI. Conveniences such as alternate GPS travel routes, alternate places for dinner, and even "amazing deals" on vacation destinations can all be very innocent . . . until they aren't. Now imagine a critically or chronically ill patient who recently has been told that their options for care and survival are limited. Suggestions for radical treatments, such as unlicensed stem cell therapies in foreign countries, can lead to terrible outcomes and not just for health but for finances also.[32] In a world where misinformation and fact are indistinguishable to a large portion of the population, automated and highly targeted disinformation at scale is nothing short of a weapon of mass destruction if unchecked.

Regulatory approaches

Given the many definitions of AI, the uncertain benefits and the incredibly broad range of possible harms from mild to severe, regulation of AI is a complex matter. Starting with the question of who should regulate AI, the traditional and default approach would be to regulate AI based upon the use case. This would have the Food and Drug Administration (FDA) regulating AI for biomedical products, the Federal Trade Commission looking into applications in trade and business, and the Federal Communications Commission looking into broader uses across the Internet and Internet service providers. This is already the case with the Department of Transportation regulating autonomous vehicle technology and unmanned aerial vehicles.

Sticking with medical products, the FDA has released several plans and draft guidances on the regulation of AI.

Preliminary approaches at FDA place authority within the FDA Centers for Devices and Radiological Health (CDRH) with the initial intent of regulating AI as software and or as software as a medical device (SaMD). From the FDA website: "The International Medical Device Regulators Forum (IMDRF) defines 'Software as a Medical Device (SaMD)' as software intended to be used for one or more medical purposes that perform these purposes without being part of a hardware medical device. FDA, under the Federal Food, Drug, and Cosmetic Act (FD&C Act) considers medical purpose as those purposes that are intended to treat, diagnose, cure, mitigate, or prevent disease or other conditions."[33] With respect to what regulatory evidence, approvals, and/or clearances are required, "When applied to AI/ML-based SaMD, the above approach would require a premarket submission to the FDA when the AI/ML software modification significantly affects device performance, or safety and effectiveness; the modification is to the device's intended use; or the modification introduces a major change to the SaMD algorithm. For a PMA-approved SaMD, a supplemental application would be required for changes that affect safety or effectiveness, such as new indications for use, new clinical effects, or significant technology modifications that affect performance characteristics." With the rationale being, that the traditional paradigm of medical device regulation was not designed for adaptive AI/ML technologies, which have the potential to adapt and optimize device performance in real-time to continuously improve health care for patients. The highly iterative, autonomous, and adaptive nature of these tools requires a new, total product lifecycle (TPLC) regulatory approach that facilitates a rapid cycle of product improvement and allows these devices to continually improve while monitoring for new threats and vulnerabilities and providing effective safeguards.

These approaches provide reasonably good coverage. The question and challenge lie in determining when something is a medical device and when it is not. Again, according to the FDA,

Non-device software functions are not subject to FDA device regulation and are not within the scope of this paper. In addition, as detailed in section 502(o) of the FD&C Act, software functions intended (1) for administrative support of a health care facility, (2) for maintaining or encouraging a healthy lifestyle, (3) to serve as electronic patient records, (4) for transferring, storing, converting formats, or displaying data, or (5) to provide certain, limited clinical decision support are not medical devices and are not subject to FDA regulation.

This is where things get dicey, especially with the hybridization between recreational health and fitness tracking and actual healthcare diagnosis, delivery, or monitoring.

In an attempt to address the explosion of software-driven medical devices, decision-support algorithms, and software-driven diagnostics, the FDA introduced the Pre-Cert pilot program in July 2017. It was specifically intended to develop a new regulatory paradigm that would focus first on the assessment of organizations that perform high-quality software design, testing, and monitoring. This proposed approach is based on demonstration of a culture of quality and organizational excellence (CQOE) and a commitment to monitoring product performance.[34] The idea here is to pre-evaluate and certify whether an organization has the necessary capabilities to deliver, manage, and control biomedical product software in this increasingly complex age. Organizations that achieve this status would be granted expedited regulatory review of their products. Companies that secure the precertification, however, may have increased postmarket surveillance and data collection obligations, with a particular emphasis on real-world data.[35]

Although precertifying innovators makes sense, there are significant concerns with how this will work in reality. First, current FDA approaches, including Pre-Cert, focus upon software quality practices, not the intent of the software, the unintended consequences, unintended bias, and similar concerns. Said differently, well-engineered software can still cause harm. Quality manufacturing is essential, but benefit risk must still be assessed. Further, this approach is untested, which has drawn the attention of legislators who feel that the FDA is lessening the focus on public safety.[36] The concerns are valid when one considers that productivity of the FDA is often measured in devices and drugs approved. However, isn't this metric, alone, contrary to the safety mission of the FDA?

In January 2019, The FDA commission and the Director of CDRH issued a press release touting, "a record year of device innovation."[37]. The statement listed the following as a claim of productivity and benefit to patients via new capabilities being available on the market: "One measure of our success in advancing device innovation is the annual number of novel, safe and effective technologies the FDA approves or clears . . . Last year, in 2018, the FDA approved 106 novel devices, surpassing the 40-year record we set in 2017 of 99 novel device approvals, and capping off eight years of steady improvement." Further the release claimed, "Our effort to promote innovation is eclipsed only by our commitment to make sure that these products are safe for patients . . . ." No metrics were provided, however, to support this "commitment to ensure safety." There are no metrics on recalls, inspections, citations, loss of clearance or approval, or any other metric as quantitative evidence of an improved, or even maintained, focus on safety. These omissions are unfortunate and must be interpreted as policy that is pro industry but not pro patient. In fact, it is simply countermessaging and evidence of the deregulation that we discussed in the 10 Toxicities chapter.

I find this lack of balance between benefits and risks problematic. Using drugs as a model because the accelerated pathways have existed longer, initial studies of accelerated pathways in cancer drug review and approval demonstrate that breakthrough-designated drugs do not provide significantly greater median PFS gains compared with non-breakthrough drugs. Studies further demonstrate that breakthrough drugs are not more likely to use a novel mechanism and that these drugs have similar rates of death as non-breakthrough drugs.[38,39] Further, the safety of drugs that have been approved via accelerated pathways is being challenged, because at least one study has shown that breakthrough drugs are clearly less safe. Ideally, these types of assessments would be the core basis of regulatory assessment. There are several ways to think about these numbers. First, if breakthrough therapies often are approved in approximately five years, versus seven years for traditional pathways, but do not offer increased efficacy or safety, what is the advantage? Further, if the safety profile of breakthrough agents is demonstrated to be lower over time, the disadvantages will be clear. Lastly, if accelerated pathways produce results that are comparable to traditional review and approval, why not apply them to every submission? If the benefit-risk calculus is the same, is the value of the accelerated pathways simply operational efficacy of the agency?

Getting back to AI, examples of accelerated review and breakthrough designation are starting to appear. In November 2019, the Food and Drug Administration provided a Breakthrough Device Designation for AI Medical Service's machine learning algorithm, which has the ability to analyze endoscopy images for potential diagnosis of gastric cancer.[40] The basis for the breakthrough designation appears to be unmet need, because most endoscopy techniques focus on colorectal cancer, which is more difficult to detect than gastric cancer. It will be interesting to see how this plays out. Clearly, if this algorithm-enhanced technique is proven to diagnose gastric cancer accurately without increasing the rates of false positives or negatives, the net benefits will outweigh the corresponding risks. The proof must include measures of performance and certainty provided by the algorithm to aide clinicians in determining whether the algorithm should be relied upon in a particular case. There have been similar FDA approvals for AI in image analysis in breast cancer, acute intracranial hemorrhage, and several aspects of pulmonary disease.[41]

The march of artificial intelligence into medicine is significant and irreversible. The benefits are becoming apparent and the risks are still largely unknown. It will require proactive effort from industry and regulators to ensure that the benefits clearly outweigh the risks, which can be especially difficult when those risks do not reside under the same lamp post as the benefits. Artificial intelligence and machine learning are simply advanced computing tools. The pros and cons, benefits and risks are inherently up to the user to decide. Tasked for good, they will move medicine forward. There is little doubt. We simply also must be prepared for when they are tasked for chaos or harm.

References

1. Marsden P. Artificial Intelligence Defined: Useful List of Popular Definitions from Business and Science. 2017, September 4. Accessed December 2019. https://digitalwellbeing.org/artificial-intelligence-defined-useful-list-of-popular-definitions-from-business-and-science/
2. Internet Society. Artificial Intelligence and Machine Learning: Policy Paper. 2017, April 18. Accessed December 2019. https://www.internetsociety.org/resources/doc/2017/artificial-intelligence-and-machine-learning-policy-paper/?gclid=CjwKCAiA8K7uBRBBEiwACOm4d5SwGgbh6SmLNsmAa-e_enyKZHqRlDMTgU4DLE8hzE1QSwETKC_4OBoCBn8QAvD_BwE
3. Parsatharathy. S. Key Differences Between Artificial Intelligence and Machine Learning. 2019, May 9. Accessed December 2019. https://towardsdatascience.com/key-differences-between-artificial-intelligence-and-machine-learning-fe637cd0deca
4. BusinessWorldIT.com. 8 Applications of Artificial Intelligence in Computer Science. 2019, January 17. Accessed December 2019. https://www.businessworldit.com/ai/applications-of-artificial-intelligence/
5. IBM. Artificial Intelligence for a Smarter Kind of Cybersecurity. AI Guide for CISOs. Accessed December 2019. https://www.ibm.com/security/artificial-intelligence
6. Narula G. Everyday Examples of Artificial. Intelligence and Machine Learning. 2019, November 21. Accessed December 2019. https://emerj.com/ai-sector-overviews/everyday-examples-of-ai/
7. Adams RL. 10 Powerful Examples of Artificial Intelligence in Use Today. 2017, January 10. Accessed December 2019. https://www.forbes.com/sites/robertadams/2017/01/10/10-powerful-examples-of-artificial-intelligence-in-use-today/#5683bf30420d
8. Razzaq A. List of AI conferences in 2019. 2019, August 12. Accessed December 2019. https://www.marktechpost.com/2019/08/12/list-of-ai-conferences-in-2019/
9. Powell A. The algorithm will see you now. *Harvard Gazette.* 2019, February 28.
10. Litjens G et al. A Survey on Deep Learning in Medical Image Analysis. *Medical Image Analysis* 2017. 42:60–88.
11. Jee C. Google's AI Is Better at Spotting Advanced Breast Cancer than Pathologists. *MIT Technology Review.* 2018, October 15.
12. Kaiser Health News. Artificial Intelligence Was as Good or Better than Doctors at Detecting Lung Cancer in Promising Study. 2019, May 21.

13. Kite-Powell J. See How Artificial Intelligence Can Improve Medical Diagnosis and Healthcare. *Forbes.* 2017, May 16.

14. Talby D. AI Will Not Replace Doctors, But It May Drastically Change Their Jobs. *Forbes.* 2019, March 15.

15. Cockburn IM, R Henderson, and S Stern. The Impact of Artificial Intelligence on Innovation: An Exploratory Analysis. National Bureau of Economic Research. 2019.

16. AI Trends Staff. White House Releases Update to National Artificial Intelligence R&D Strategic Plan. 2019, June 27. Accessed December 2019. https://www.aitrends.com/ai-in-government/white-house-releases-update-to-national-artificial-intelligence-rd-strategic-plan/

17. U.S. FDA. Software as a Medical Device (SaMD). 2018, December 4. Accessed December 2019. https://www.fda.gov/medical-devices/digital-health/software-medical-device-samd

18. Hayner C. 36 of the Best Movies About AI, Ranked. 2018, January 18. Accessed December 2019. https://www.zdnet.com/pictures/15-of-the-best-movies-about-ai-ranked/13/

19. Marr B. Is Artificial Intelligence Dangerous? 6 AI Risks Everyone Should Know About. *Forbes.* 2018, November 18.

20. NS wiki. Warm War Definition. Accessed December 2019. http://archive.nswiki.org/index.php?title=Warm_War

21. Locker L. China's Terrifying "Social Credit" Surveillance System Is Expanding. *Fast Company.* 2018, April 24.

22. Buolamwini J. Artificial Intelligence Has a Problem with Gender and Racial Bias. *Here's How to Solve It.* 2019, February 7.

23. Faggella D. Risks of AI—What Researchers Think is Worth Worrying About. 2019, January 31. Accessed December 2019. https://emerj.com/ai-market-research/artificial-intelligence-risk/

24. Sullivan HR, and SJ Schweikart. Are Current Tort Liability Doctrines Adequate for Addressing Injury Caused by AI? 2019, February. Accessed January 2020. https://journalofethics.ama-assn.org/article/are-current-tort-liability-doctrines-adequate-addressing-injury-caused-ai/2019-02

25. Anderson A, and SL Anderson. How Should AI Be Developed, Validated, and Implemented in Patient Care? 2019, February. Accessed January 2020.

26. Scripps Research. Eric Topol Pens Book on Artificial Intelligence in Medicine. 2019, March 12. Accessed October 2019. https://www.scripps.edu/news-and-events/press-room/2019/20190312-topol-deep-medicine.html

27. Hicks J. Understanding Relative Value Units. Very Well Health. 2020, January 20. Accessed January 2020. https://www.verywellhealth.com/rvu-physician-compensation-based-on-productivity-2317026

28. Owasp.org. What is Attack Surface and Why is it Important? Accessed December 2019. https://cheatsheetseries.owasp.org/cheatsheets/Attack_Surface_Analysis_Cheat_Sheet.html

29. Irwin L. How Long Does It Take to Detect a Cyberattack? IT Governance USA. 2019, March 14. Accessed December 2019. https://www.itgovernanceusa.com/blog/how-long-does-it-take-to-detect-a-cyber-attack

30. Finlayson SG et al. Adversarial Attacks Against Medical Deep Learning Systems. Accessed December 2019. https://arxiv.org/pdf/1804.05296.pdf

31. Mind Matters. AI Social Media Could Totally Manipulate You. 2018, November. 26. Accessed December 2019. https://mindmatters.ai/2018/11/ai-social-media-could-totally-manipulate-you/

32. Kowalcyzk L. He Went Abroad for Stem Cell Treatment and Now He Is a Cautionary Tale. *Boston Globe.* 2016, June 22.

33. U.S. FDA. Proposed Regulatory Framework for Modifications to Artificial Intelligence and Machine Learning-based Software as a Medical Device (SaMD). Accessed January 2020. https://www.fda.gov/media/122535/download

34. U.S. FDA. Developing Software Pre-Certification Program: A Working Model. 2018, June. Accessed December 2019. https://www.fda.gov/media/113802/download

35. McDermott W, and McDermott E. To Market, To Market: FDA's Digital Health Precertification Program. *JDSUPRA*. 2019, September 18.

36. Landi H. Sen. Elizabeth Warren, Top Democrats Continue Scrutiny of FDA's Pre-Certification Pilot for Digital Health. *FierceHealthcare*. 2019, October 30.

37. U.S. FDA. FDA Statement: Statement from FDA Commissioner Scott Gottlieb, M.D., and Jeff Shuren, M.D., Director of the Center for Devices and Radiological Health, on a Record Year for Device Innovation. 2019, January 28.

38. Hwang TJ et al. Efficacy, Safety, and Regulatory Approval of Food and Drug Administration-Designated Breakthrough and Nonbreakthrough Cancer Medicines. *Journal of Clinical Oncology* 2018. 36(18):1805–1812.

39. Radcliffe S. Is the "Breakthrough Therapy" Process Putting Dangerous Drugs on Store Shelves? *Healthline*. 2018, April 17.

40. Parmar A. Japanese Firm's AIAlgorithm for Gastric Cancer gets FDA's Breakthrough Device Designation. *Med City News*. 2019, November 11.

41. Carfagno J. 5 FDA Approved Uses of AI in Healthcare. Docwire. 2019, July 28. Accessed December 2019. https://www.docwirenews.com/docwire-pick/future-of-medicine-picks/fda-approved-uses-of-ai-in-healthcare/

19

Virtual Health Assistants

One of the more anticipated capabilities of digital health are digital health assistants. Alexa, Siri, and Cortana have clearly changed the way that people interact with computers and devices. From voice commands directing functionality on a mobile phone, to voice commands for "smart" devices within homes, virtual assistants have enabled hands-free operation and offered convenience and safety. According to *Lifewire*, "Virtual assistants like these can do everything from answer questions, tell jokes, play music, and control items in your home such as lights, thermostat, door locks, and smart home devices. They can respond to many voice commands, send text messages, make phone calls, set up reminders. Anything you do on your phone; you can probably ask your virtual assistant to do for you . . . ." These devices are truly impressive and are fulfilling the promise that digital technologies will transform our lives.

In health care, there is significant expectation and hope riding on virtual assistants. The market potential had been estimated at almost $2 billion by 2015. As we discussed earlier, there is a range of current and future applications starting with the mundane, such as automated chatbots for medical appointment scheduling, to the far more complex, as in, "the algorithm will see you now." The needs driving the virtual assistant market are driving other elements of health care; an aging population, a shortage of healthcare professionals, increasing complexity in the management of chronic diseases, and an enthusiastic and well-funded technology sector promising breakthrough solutions.

Currently, the primary use cases mirror other market segments and focus on speech recognition and talk-to-text functionalities. Health care application of these use cases includes medical transcription, voice-to-text functionality to ease electronic health record () usage pains, search, and scheduling. That said, true adoption, that is, the actual and full replacement of current systems and processes has been slow. Everything from the complexity of medical jargon, the concern and consequences of mistakes and errors, even the background noise in many medical settings pose a challenge for current technologies. This has created the need for "smarter" listening, specifically for devices and capabilities designed to mitigate the healthcare setting-specific challenges. For example, an application from Sopris Health, trained via many

Digital Health. Eric D. Perakslis and Martin Stanley, Oxford University Press (2021). © Oxford University Press.
DOI: 10.1093/oso/9780197503133.003.0019

hours of learning on audio from actual clinician visit conversations not only converts speech to text but also creates a doctor's note.[3] Being able to discern the medically relevant portions of any conversation is the machine-enhanced learning behind these important capabilities, but responsibility for the accuracy of the information still lies with the clinician, which is a barrier to adoption. This type of justifiable concern leads to an all too common problem of healthcare systems today, unintentional redundancy.

When considering digital transformation of any process or system, comprehensive testing and rigorous change management are essential. These tests, however, are often less than fully satisfying to concerned and responsible healthcare professionals. The result can be dabbling and prolonged pilots where multiple systems are run in parallel for longer than anticipated periods of time. Sometimes this is unavoidable, most commonly because the newer technology offers only a partial solution. This results in the necessity to maintain the old while trying to implement the new, essentially doubling the systems burden on groups that were actually seeking to reduce time spent. The ability to design technology evaluation pilots well is one of the greatest unmet needs in digital transformation and will continue to be problematic until organizations evolve to the understanding that successful digital transformation requires a new type of cooperative methodology that spans engineering, science, compliance, and medicine.[4]

Privacy issues

Continuing with that *Live Wire* quote, "even better, virtual assistants can learn over time and get to know your habits and preferences, so they're always getting smarter. Using artificial intelligence (AI), virtual assistants can understand natural language, recognize faces, identify objects, and communicate with other smart devices and software." There are significant ethical and privacy issues here to unpack. The benefit is, of course, convenience, but the risks are less clear.

Starting with the fact that digital assistants recognize faces and voices, it is important to understand that facial recognition and voice recognition are forms of biometric identity. Biometrics can be generally described as the ability to recognize or even uniquely identify individuals based upon physical characteristics. To date, in the United States, there is no privacy law regulating the use of biometric identity, although biometric identity is covered under the Global Data Protection Regulations (GDPR) in Europe. Practically, this means that, because AI is learning from every interaction, the machine is building a complex and multidimensional model of each individual who interacts with it and that these models evolve to better specificity over time. Now take it one step further and consider that all these assistants must be connected to the Internet to perform most functions. The result is that Siri, Alexa, or Cortana are aggregating massive data profiles of each user. Further, a user really has no idea with whom, when, or how the information is being shared. Sounds Orwellian, I know, but data transfers happen all the time. One piece in the *Guardian* reported that contractors for Apple regularly hear confidential medical information, drug deals, and recordings of couples having sex, as part of their job providing quality control.[5] These users were unaware that they were being recorded and that the recording left their homes. Although Apple suspended the "grading program" that led to these disclosures, there is no way to know what other programs still exist.

Even without such programs, the imperfections in digital assistants pose risk. For example, manufacturers insist that these devices only listen when triggered, usually by a phrase such as "Hey Siri," but can they prove it? Do we really know? Can they be hacked? Further, because the devices are always actively listening and awaiting activation and because speech recognition is imperfect, devices can be accidentally triggered and can be active for prolonged periods of times without the "user" knowing. Interestingly, tech experts feel that the public should be savvier. "People have a somewhat unrealistic expectation that these assistants will by magic just get better eventually, that they can do machine learning and get better on their own . . . but human intervention is still important," according to Carolina Milanesi.[6] She is referring to the fact that human intervention, specifically human listening, is often needed to keep these assistants running and for research and development (R&D). Indeed, consumers must be more aware.

Lastly, it is interesting to consider how the HIPAA compliance of digital assistants impact privacy. In April 2019, Amazon announced a version of Alexa that is "HIPPA compliant." Specifically, this meant that there was a new version available for applications that are subject to the data privacy and security requirements of HIPAA. This new version of Alexa, more specifically, the Alexa Skills Kit, was available to a limited number of developers by invitation only.[7] The major change is that Alexa could now be used by computing applications that manage personal health information (PHI). It is important to note, however, that this in no way meant that the commercially available Alexa versions for home use were now suitable for sensitive health data, although many perceived it this way. Clearly a great step forward, but, as we have already discussed, the actual privacy protections of HIPAA are limited and outdated.

Security issues

It is important to understand that these platforms have capabilities similar to active surveillance. According to *The Atlantic*, "When saved queries—and often, associated location data—are connected to user accounts, they can paint a very accurate picture of users' habits, travels, and preferences . . . But the resulting data-portraits are also available to law enforcement officers who come knocking with a subpoena in hand . . . —and they can be stolen by hackers who gain access to sensitive servers."[8]

How far should or could these devices go in health care with respect to balancing convenience and physical security? What if a device hears a threat, an altercation, or even breaking glass or sounds of a scuffle? Should they automatically call the police or an ambulance? Law enforcement is using intentional and unintentional recordings because high-profile cases ranging from burglary to double murder have involved subpoena of digital assistant data.[9,10] Regardless, digital assistants have been shown to be a hackers' dream as they have been turned into listening devices, used as access points to enter other computers in the home, and shown to be vulnerable to tampering via sounds inaudible to humans.[11]

Security-enhancing features are also possible with digital assistants. The MedicAlert Foundation has been in operation since 1956 and focuses on the secure storage and transmission of vital healthcare information between patients and healthcare providers and emergency medical services.[12] Having better data, readily available in an emergency has clear benefit, especially for the elderly, the infirm, or the disabled. Similarly, these technologies can enable remote caregivers to be in closer touch with those under their care. The cost of this convenience is privacy and the trade-offs must be well understood. An interesting use case is to employ surveillance as medical monitoring. For example, University of Washington researchers recently published a study in which they taught Alexa and two other devices—an iPhone 5s and a Samsung Galaxy S4—to listen for so-called agonal breathing, the distinct gasping sounds that are an early warning sign in about half of all cardiac arrests. These devices correctly identified agonal breathing in 97% of instances, while registering a false positive only 0.2% of the time.[13]

The ultimate question is how to balance the benefits and risks of digital assistants? For healthy, normal people who are free from chronic disease and carry very little medical risk, the privacy and security concerns should tip the scales toward caution. For the infirm, the balance may be a closer call. Let's look at some use cases.

In September 2018, Amazon filed a patent for a version of Alexa that can recognize illness or emotion, using voice recognition and analysis.[14] This means that Alexa can tell if you are coming down with a cold. Very cool, but what does the assistant do with the data? Is the information useful diagnostic information that can be organically integrated into telehealth delivery? Is it used by Amazon to recommend products? Should it suggest medications or medication reminders? These elements are all under review and highlight the inherent risks of unsupervised health care. Another area of interesting progress is diabetes management. In April 2018, Amazon and Merck & Co., Inc. jointly started the Alexa Diabetes Challenge with a $250,000 prize pot. Wellpepper emerged as the winner with its Sugarpod, a clinically validated and Alexa-enabled digital platform for diabetes management. With Sugarpod, Alexa is able to help diabetic patients manage their treatments and monitor progress effectively. According to the chief-executive-officer (CEO) of Wellpepper, "Sugarpod helps newly diagnosed people with type 2 diabetes integrate new information and routines into the fabric of their daily lives to self-manage, connect to care, and avoid complications." This is a solid example of utility in the management of chronic diseases. Diabetes management has always been challenging. Remembering to check blood sugar, correlating blood sugar readings with dietary choices, and titrating insulin and/or other medication doses has always been iterative and trial and error. Having better data and ready guidance is surely beneficial. Similar solutions are available for blood pressure monitoring and Parkinson's disease, with many more on the way. All that said, opportunities for digital assistants revolve around automating search via voice.[16] Everything from medication dosages to parking information at a local care center can be made available via voice and the digital breadcrumbs mirror those resulting from traditional web searches enriched by the associated biometric data.

The surveillance and privacy risks of extensive use of virtual assistants are quite clear. Specifically, these devices are recoding biometric data that can be used to uniquely identify a user with very high precision, and this is occurring unbeknownst to most users. Further, the dialogue history contains location data, frequently visited places, information about diet, exercise, medication, symptomology, and frequent contacts, much of which could be considered personal health information. The greatest opportunities in health care appear to be targeted health application built using the HIPAA compliant toolkits, when available, such as with Amazon Alexa.

Ideally, privacy and security standards for virtual assistants will be created that ensure when the devices are on or off, encrypt all captured information end-to-end, and provide specific guidance on exactly what types of use are permittable by technology suppliers with consent and without consent. Earlier we reviewed integrated approaches to security and privacy that could do just that. Lastly, the information or advice provided by these devices is never going to be better than the sources they draw upon to fulfill queries. Users must understand that they are not speaking with a wise or sentient being. They are speaking with a simple Google search and must apply caution and good sense when considering the answers.

An idealized opportunity to balance benefits and risks

As speech recognition by virtual assistants only improves with use, the ideal solution for patients and health care may be via combined privacy and security education in the form of voice recognition training models. Most virtual assistants already include voice training modules and capabilities designed to improve accuracy and utility.[17] Similar programs could be designed that walk patients through privacy and security tips instead of random sentences or sentences designed to practice articulation across a range of words and sounds. Indeed, these courses could be designed to deliver just as much vocal variety as delivered through topical tutorials. Further, in clinical trials for complex chronic disease regimens, such approaches may improve adherence and data quality while minimizing privacy and security risks via sound awareness training.

References

1. McLaughlin M. What a Virtual Assistant Is and How It Works. Lifewire. 2019, December 2. Accessed December 2019. https://www.lifewire.com/virtual-assistants-4138533
2. Pennic J. Healthcare Virtual Assistant Market to Reach $1.76. Billion by 2025. *HIT Consultant.* 2019, August 23.
3. Molteni M. Does Your Doctor Need a Voice Assistant? *Wired.* 2018, May 1.
4. Perakslis ED. Strategies for Delivering Value from Digital Technology Transformation. *Nature Reviews. Drug Discovery* 2017. 16(2):71–72. doi:10.1038/nrd.2016.265
5. Hern A. Apple Contractors Regularly Hear Confidential Details on Siri Recordings. *The Guardian.* 2019, July 26.
6. Lever R. Privacy Missteps Cast Cloud over Digital Assistants. Tech Explore. 2019, August 3. Accessed October 2019. https://techxplore.com/news/2019–08-privacy-missteps-cloud-digital.html
7. Treloar N. Alexa Is Now HIPAA-Eligible, So What's Next for Healthcare? *HIT Consultant.* 2019, April 5.
8. Waddell K. The Privacy Problem with Digital Assistants. *The Atlantic.* 2016, May 24.
9. Dreier N. Alexa Helps Solve House Break-In Mystery. *AJC.* 2017, July 27.

10. Seidel J. Amazon Echo Recordings May Hold Key to New Hampshire Murders. 2018, November 12. Accessed December 2019. https://www.news.com.au/technology/home-entertainment/audio/home-assistant-smart-speaker-recordings-may-hold-key-to-new-hampshire-murders/news-story/70271a080cfa3bf953eecd912204e225

11. Lemos R. Five Ways Digital Assistants Pose Security Threats to the Home, Office. 2018, July 2. Eweek. Accessed November 2019. https://www.eweek.com/security/five-ways-digital-assistants-pose-security-threats-in-home-office

12. Wikipedia. Medic Alert. Accessed October 2019. https://en.wikipedia.org/wiki/MedicAlert

13. Rae-Dupree J. Doctor Alexa Will See You Now: Is Amazon Primed to Come to Your Rescue? *FierceHealthcare*. 2019, July 29.

14. Spanu A. Amazon's New Alexa Will Know If Someone Is Sick Just By Listening To Their Voice. *Healthcare Weekly*. 2018, October 10.

15. Alexa Diabetes Challenge. And oor winner is . . . Sugarpod by Wellpepper! Alexa Diabetes Challenge Blog. 2017, October 16. Accessed November 2019. http://www.alexadiabeteschallenge.com/winner-sugarpod-wellpepper/

16. Bora P. Alexa in Healthcare: 17 Real Use Cases You Should Know About. DAP. 2019, March 6. Accessed October 2019. https://www.digitalauthority.me/resources/alexa-in-healthcare/

17. Hoffman C. How to Train Siri, Cortana and Alexa to Understand Your Voice Better. How-to Geek. 2017, June 20. Accessed October 2019. https://www.howtogeek.com/231329/how-to-train-siri-cortana-and-google-to-understand-your-voice-better/

20
Wearables

According to a history of wearables infographic published by Phillips, the earliest recorded instance of a health wearable is attributed to a sketch of a pedometer by Leonardo DaVinci from as early as 1472.[1] Other significant development stages include: the first pedometer, the Tomish Meter, in the United States introduced by Thomas Jefferson in 1788; the introduction of the polygraph in 1921; the first wearable hearing aid in 1938; the first fully digital pacemaker in 2001; and the Nike and iPod system launched in 2006. After that, the timeline is densely packed with new products and capabilities, a true explosion of growth. To the Phillips timeline, I would add the release of the Holter monitor for remote cardio-physiological monitoring in 1962, previously detailed developments in pulse oximetry in the late 1980s, the first GPS-enabled wristwatch introduced by Casio in 1999, and the launch of the first Fitbit in 2009.[2]

One of the more interesting perspectives from which the development of wearable technologies can be considered is by contrasting wellness and medicine, which are often conflated and referred to as "health" by purveyors of these technologies. Several important lines of demarcation must be understood. For example, heart rate is a foundational vital sign and is measured and recorded during most clinical encounters regardless of whether the encounter is a periodic "well" visit physical exam or a "sick" visit intended to diagnose and/or treat an injury or illness. Although it is clear that tracking heart rate is a valuable tool in measuring fitness while exercising, there is not yet significant evidence that shows continuous heart rate tracking has any health benefits otherwise.[3] Indeed, some clinicians feel that this type of personal monitoring can cause more harm than good as heart rate fluctuates constantly and overinterpretation is a likely outcome. We also know that this extensive self-monitoring can promote cyberchondria. This is where things get dicey. For example, it is well known that people who weigh themselves regularly tend to lose or maintain body weight more consistently than those who don't and that healthy body weight often reduces risks of cardiovascular disease and some cancers. Does this then mean that it is credible for a bathroom scale manufacturer to claim that their product lowers cancer risk? Most would see this as a

Digital Health. Eric D. Perakslis and Martin Stanley, Oxford University Press (2021). © Oxford University Press.
DOI: 10.1093/oso/9780197503133.003.0020

stretch, yet this is exactly the situation we see today with the Apple Watch and other "health" wearables that are being hyped as medical solutions.

Further, the wearables landscape is extremely complex and crowded. There are dozens of readily available consumer grade devices that serve as some form of connected technology. One distinguishing factor is whether they work fully independently or whether they must be digitally tethered in some way to a smartphone. Most of the higher-end wearables fit into this latter category because the computing power is greatly enhanced, while simultaneously reducing the computing storage and processing needs on the actual watch, ring, or other form factor. This also greatly increases attack surface, as we have discussed. Given the diversity of this rapidly changing market, we will not review the hundreds and hundreds of physical devices, associated apps, and corresponding advertorial and medic claims and hype. Instead, we will use the most common exemplar of the wearables market, the Apple Watch, as a case study of the opportunities and issues surrounding these technologies.

Case study: Irregular heartbeat "approval" for the Apple Watch threat-based interpretation of Apple clearance letter

One of the growing pains of digital health is the proper understanding of nomenclature and language. In particular, the terms FDA "approved" and FDA "cleared" often are used interchangeably, especially by the lay press, but they are actually very different in meaning. The Food and Drug Administration (FDA) defines approved medical devices as those devices for which the FDA has approved a premarket approval (PMA) application or a Humanitarian Device Exemption (HDE) application. This review and approval process is for Class III medical devices (the ones with the highest risk) and involves a more rigorous review than the 510(k) review process. FDA cleared devices are those that FDA has determined to be substantially equivalent to (similar to) another legally marketed device. A premarket notification submission is referred to as a 510(k) and must be submitted to the FDA to review and provide clearance.[5] In January 2019, I published a *British Medical Journal Blog* piece on this topic using the clearance letter for the irregular heartbeat feature of the Apple Watch.[6] Within this piece I dissected exactly what the FDA Clearance letter stated and did not state.

First, and most importantly, the letter clearly articulated that these devices do not yet have clinical grade accuracy or precision. The FDA response letter also identifies a number of risks associated with using the device, such as false negatives, false positives, misinterpretation, and potential overreliance on the device.[7] Although the FDA letter highlights these points, they were immediately lost in the media frenzy and hype that followed the announcement of the FDA clearance. First of all, many of these stories declared the watch had been "approved" for arrythmia detection. Statements that were wrong on both points. There is also a difference between irregular heartbeat detection and actual arrhythmia diagnostics. Not only were these important differences lost to the press, medical luminaries on Twitter and other social media were sharing these inaccurate pieces and touting the advancements for patients. A clear case of medical misinformation!

There are several important issues here to unpack. First, as discussed earlier, the FDA regulates the tools employed by health care but does not regulate health care. Unfortunately, this means that many clinicians have a poor understanding of the FDA. They don't understand exactly what the agency does or how it does it. Digital health is bringing this to the surface. Second, this example shows the massive gaps in expertise, diligence, and rigor between the technology press and the peer-reviewed medical literature. It is not that doctors do not seek out quality sources of truth on digital tools, it is that those examples are few and far between compared to the media hype engines.

The Apple Watch clearance represented a major lost opportunity to consider and address the issues and best practices around privacy and security. Further, medical wearable devices are themselves biometric data collection and transmission devices, which greatly amplify privacy risks. Modern biometrics, such as facial recognition, fingerprints, gait, iris and retinal scanning, touch typing, voice recognition, heart rate/rhythm, and others are the basis of next-generation identity management technologies. In short, most digital health sensors are also biometric measurement and transmission devices. Just as a DNA sequence can be used to provide important medical insights, that same sequence also can be used uniquely to identify an individual. Biometric identifiers such as facial recognition are especially difficult to secure and protect because they can be captured without notice, are easily tampered with, and are easily compared to faces scraped from the web and social media sites; therefore they can be easily weaponized. None of these data streams are explicitly covered under HIPAA, but they are protected under General Data Protection Regulations (GDPR) in Europe. The question is whether these regulations and enforcement will be able to keep up with the speed of development and implementation of these technologies.[9] GDPR is more comprehensive than HIPAA and closes some of the HIPAA loopholes. Under GDPR, biometric data is explicitly covered under "special categories of personal data" and can only be processed and used under explicit consent or other clearly described circumstances.[10]

In terms of security, we know health care is a high-value cybertarget and will continue to face persistent threats.[11] Devices are at risk of being hacked, and modern smartphones have the potential to be highly advanced surveillance devices in the hands of determined adversaries. According to a recent report from the U.S. Department of Homeland Security (DHS) on mobile device security, mobile devices and connected accessories are easy to lose or steal, often connected to unsecured public wireless networks, and are subject to an extensive range of cyberattacks that include geolocation disclosure, tampering, denial of service, identity and data disclosure, phishing and device hijacking.[12] Geolocation disclosure is especially troubling because the threats here go beyond the financial and reputational attacks we have witnessed to date. We must understand that by mixing health and location data we open up an entirely new domain of privacy and physical threats. Location data is currently unregulated and enables deep surveillance of individuals' activity, location, and habits without their notice.[13] In conclusion, the exclusion of any form of cybersecurity guidance, monitoring requirements, or preventative controls within the Apple clearance letter was a huge lost opportunity to not only protect users but to set precedent in a rapidly emerging consumer marketplace.

To believe the hype and market forecasts for consumer and medical wearables is to assume that, soon, most humans will have a device on their person that connects to the Internet by voice, is capable of transmitting biometric identity and location information, and is an amplifier of the total attack surface of each person's smartphone. From the standpoint of benefit risk, this can be an amazing opportunity for individuals with many types of chronic and degenerative diseases to have some direct personal connectivity to the inherent diagnostic and, possibly, treatment opportunities. For those who are healthy, these devices offer many ways to stay healthy and even improve athleticism and mood, but all of this does come at the price of sacrificing privacy, security (physical and cyber), and autonomy. Clearly a case of caveat emptor that should be the careful focus of health regulators given the clear and persistent threats involved.

References

1. Phillips. Infographic: The History of Wearables. Phillips News Center. 2016, September 29. Accessed December 2019. https://www.philips.com/a-w/about/news/archive/future-health-index/articles/20160929-infographic-history-wearables.html

2. News18 Staff. The World's First Wristwatch with Built-In GPS. 2016, May 15. Accessed October 2019. https://www.news18.com/news/tech/the-worlds-first-wristwatch-with-built-in-gps-1243256.html

3. Rettner R. New Heart Rate Trackers: Is Knowing Your Pulse Useful? Live Science. 2013, December 23. Accessed October 2019. https://www.livescience.com/42132-heart-rate-activity-tracker-useful.html

4. Elektra Labs. Digital Measures Atlas. Accessed January 2020. https://elektralabs.com/solutions

5. U.S. FDA. What Is the Difference Between Cleared and Approved? 2019, April 9. Accessed January 2019. https://www.fda.gov/medical-devices/resources-you-medical-devices/consumers-medical-devices#What_is_the_difference_between_Cleared_and_Approved_

6. Perakslis E. Protecting Patient Privacy and Security While Exploiting the Utility of Next Generation Digital Health Wearables. *BMJ Blog*. 2019, January 18.

7. U.S. FDA. Response to De Novo request for classification of the Irregular Rhythm Notification Feature. Angela C. Krueger Deputy Director, Engineering and Science Review Office of Device Evaluation Center for Devices and Radiological Health. September 11, 2018.

8. Cohen IG, and MM Mello. HIPAA and Protecting Health Information in the 21st Century. *JAMA* 2018. 320(3): 231–232.

9. Owen D. Should We Be Worried About Computerized Facial Recognition? *The New Yorker*. 2018, December 17.

10. https://gdpr-info.eu/art-9-gdpr/

11. Jarrett MP. Cybersecurity—A Serious Patient Care Concern. *JAMA* 2017. 318(14):1319–1320.

12. U.S. Department of Homeland Security. Study on Mobile Device Security. Accessed December 2019. https://www.dhs.gov/sites/default/files/publications/DHS%20Study%20on%20Mobile%20Devic

13. Harris R. Your Apps Know Where You Were Last Night and Are Not Keeping It a Secret. *New York Times*. 2018, December 10.

PART 5

THE FUTURE OF DIGITAL HEALTH BENEFIT-RISK ASSESSMENT AND MANAGEMENT

21

Five Mitigations for the 10 Toxicities

Awareness and education on new models of risk

The primary purpose of this book was to raise awareness and to educate on the new and emerging risks that accompany digital health. Because the risks are newly identified in many cases, we cannot offer formal solutions given that most are works in progress. We hope that awareness and education will serve as a foundation on which solid solutions can be built. Recalling the cyberrisk equation as a mental model,

Risk = Threat * Vulnerability * Impact * Likelihood.

We propose applying an enhanced version of this equation for digital health risk by modification of the Vulnerability factor as follows to account for the quantifiable parts of the 10 Toxicities:

Vulnerability = $I(Vt + Vhi)$

Vt is defined as traditional technology/human factors vulnerabilities. Vhi is defined as the specific physical, psychosocial, or socioeconomic vulnerabilities of a patient based upon the 10 Toxicities. In the equation, I is defined as scalar that is greater than or equal to 1, that relates to the increase in attack surface vulnerability of a healthcare intervention. The resulting risk equation is:

Risk = Threat * I(Vt + Vhi) * Impact * Likelihood.

Considering the specifics within the context of an example, let's compare the relative risks of monitoring a patient for atrial fibrillation (Afib) using a modern, Internet-connected, Holter monitor, and the recently cleared Apple Watch abnormal heart rate detection feature. As it is a current standard of care, we will assign I = 1 for the Holter monitor. We will also assume that the patient populations are of equal risk from the standpoint of medical

Digital Health. Eric D. Perakslis and Martin Stanley, Oxford University Press (2021). © Oxford University Press.
DOI: 10.1093/oso/9780197503133.003.0021

frailty, socioeconomic status, and other elements of the 10 Toxicities except cybersecurity, physical security, and privacy, so:

Vhi-holter = Vhi-applewatch.

Let's also assume that *Vt-holter* = V*t-applewatch*, just for the sake of simplicity. The I term for each is significantly different. In the case of the Holter Monitor, the device is sealed, records data over a shorter time span, and is not connected to a prolific digital ecosystem. The Apple Watch, by comparison, has a much larger exposure footprint due to its relatively complex operating system which can be updated with new features, hardware, built-in communication system, and connected eco system (iPhone, app store, etc.). The Apple Watch can be connected to bluetooth, Wi-Fi, and the cellular network, all of which increase cyberexposure and vulnerability. Further, the device tracks the location of the user, increasing physical security vulnerability. As we've previously discussed, these types of vulnerabilities compound and cascade. Anywhere the patient connects the Apple Watch to Wi-Fi, the attack surface is increased. For comparison, assigning an arbitrary integer to each, we see that I-*applewatch* = 5*I-*holter,* meaning that the vulnerability component for the Apple Watch is 5 times greater.

These are the kinds of considerations that must become part of the dialogue among those who build, prescribe, and utilize digital health solutions. The intent is not to slow or restrict progress, but to communicate and consider the corresponding risks that are quantifiable and qualitatively understood but not yet fully quantified. Education and awareness of these risks should happen at every possible level and opportunity. Just as a clinician warns of possible drug side effects, they should mention cyber, privacy, and other risks when a patient asks their opinion on the latest "health-tech" wearable. New language and strategies are needed to deal with misinformation, cyberchondria, and even the physical security risks posed by GPS-enabled health technologies. For example, when advertising or prescribing the health benefits of the Apple Watch abnormal heart rate detection feature, perhaps the fact that a patient's personal health information, identity, and anonymity *may* be at greater risk should be included in this notice. Those designing clinical trials must account for these additional hazards within the risk management framework of each trial. Digital health entrepreneurs would be best served by accounting for and building risk reduction into their products and marketing strategies. Again, the point is not to fear digital health tools, but to apply them when the benefit clearly outweighs the risks.

A new regulatory paradigm is needed

Digital health continues to be heralded as a solution for many healthcare ills, but the current regulatory response is underpowered and risks patient safety and autonomy. As we have discussed throughout this book, cyberthreats and other inherent threats of healthcare digitization are real and diverse, complex and prolific. They are even more concerning when the unintended consequences of social media dependency, medical misinformation, and the other toxicities of digital health are considered.[1] New regulatory approaches based upon quantifiable benefit-risks of cybersecurity, medical device safety, privacy, and artificial intelligence are needed.

With respect to cybersecurity and privacy, according to the Privacy Rights Clearinghouse Database, there have been 4,663 data breaches in the United States since 2005, with some 3,211 occurring since 2013.[2] During that same 2013–present time frame, the FDA has issued nine Cybersecurity Safety Communications.[3] While the FDA safety communications were specific to medical devices and the larger list of more than 3,200 is not (it includes hospitals, health plans, government agencies, and many similar types of facilities), the fact that many hospitals do not recognize when, or ever discover, that medical devices have been hacked, it is a sound assumption that the occurrence is far larger than the nine instances communicated by the FDA.[4] Further, the fragmentation of current and proposed privacy legislation across various state and federal agencies makes determining proper regulatory oversight of new forms of digital tools and services an intractable debate.

Benefit-risk determination precedes regulatory filings, and the traditional arbiters, ethics review committees and/or institutional review boards are already underpowered to address emerging technologies. Interestingly, significant debate exists on the utility of algorithms and other quantitative methodologies in benefit-risk assessment.[5,6] If ethics committees and regulators are hesitant to utilize quantitative models and algorithms in assessing medical products, how are these groups expected to assess benefits and risks of these technologies themselves?

With respect to medical device deregulation, significant gaps threaten patient safety. The FDA continues to exempt more and more devices, such as blood glucose meters, from premarket notification requirements.[7] Statements such as, "Non-device software functions are not subject to FDA device regulation and are not within the scope . . . ," highlight the fact that few digital tools fit comfortably within the traditional definitions of medical devices, or other preexisting regulatory classifications. Another widening loophole is treating algorithms like software. For example, recent writing from the FDA primarily discusses best practices for software development, management, and change control but not bias and other well documented hazards.[8] Similarly, all algorithms cannot be treated as if they are equal, carry equal risk, or offer equal benefit. Machine-learning algorithms often cannot be understood by humans, and, therefore, cannot be regulated simply as software or human-created algorithms that are readable.[9] Lastly, there are additive effects of digital tools that are not considered within current regulatory approaches. Using attack surface as an example, the additive effects of each additional Internet-connected device to the attack surface in any case is readily identifiable and calculable yet not discussed within current regulatory approaches. Ignoring attack surface, the increase in attack surface caused by digital health, and the risks posed by an increased attack surface is simply irresponsible.

Create a dedicated digital health center at the Food and Drug Administration

The precedent of creating a separate Food and Drug Administration (FDA) center for products of similar purpose but highly varied complexity already exists at FDA given that drugs and biologics are regulated differently via CDER and CBER. According to the FDA, "In contrast to most drugs that are chemically synthesized, and their structure is known, most biologics are complex mixtures that are not easily identified or characterized."[10] This type of distinction is exactly what separates traditional human-developed software and machine-generated algorithms. Machine-generated algorithms are not humanly readable in the ways that human-generated software is, and necessitate different approaches for regulation. It is not that the good people within the Centers for Devices and Radiological Health (CDRH), the FDA desk responsible for medical devices are not trying. The issue is that shoehorning radically different technologies into older product models is inadequate.

First, consumer notification must be modernized to ensure actionability. In examining the FDA cybersecurity safety communications referenced earlier, the actions suggested are not as consumer friendly as, "Don't eat the lettuce in the pink bag." These communications call for patients to contact providers, who may or may not know if any given patient's device is affected; for providers to contact manufacturers; for providers to perform updates of firmware and other complex tasks. Although each of these alerts is technically correct, is the audience ready and able to respond? Clearly, the magnitude of the impacts of not doing this right warrants deep consideration and a fresh approach.

Next, create new regulatory classifications based upon new approaches for assessing, determining, and codifying benefit risks. For example, are three medical device classifications adequate for digital health? Given all we have discussed, can all or even most digital tools be classified accurately as high, medium, or low risk? Application of the concepts of attack surface demonstrate that the risks posed by Internet-connected digital devices varies depending on where and how they are used and the nature of connectivity. Although nontrivial, moving from a three-tier classification model to a four- or even a five-tier model would facilitate greatly needed granularity to codify the risks of these new tools.

Modernize the safety net. The surveillance net that captures, assesses, and acts upon adverse events for traditional medical devices is simply inadequate for the digital age. Instead of a process of mostly voluntary reports flowing into federal agencies, we need a real-time surveillance net that constantly monitors threats and searches for events far more actively. Done adequately, this would look much more like a threat operations center one would expect to see in an IT command center than a traditional public health or medical safety office. Warnings must be modernized to communicate threats accurately but in ways that are actionable by patients, providers, and institutions.

Quantify benefit risk. As medicine, risk, and benefit are all math-based and quantifiable, regulators cannot continue to assess and determine benefit risk with solely qualitative methods. These approaches fall short of adequately determining benefit risk, especially the important network effects of benefit risk that can be risk multipliers as we have shown. There are a multitude of available models. Instead of treating quantitative methods as peripheral to benefit-risk determination, they must be improved and adopted as fundamental table stakes.

Improve premarket procedures. The current trend of device deregulation is occurring at a time of great change and emergence of a multitude of new and not yet understood threats. Stronger premarket approval processes can be simplified, however, if fundamental changes are made to current trends. For example, the current default for the Internet connectivity of new health devices is the "on" position. If the default were switched to the "off" position, new digital health tools working within this approach would likely be determined to be lower risk and benefit from accelerated marketing authorizations.

We must advocate for the adequate and proper regulation of digital health products. The threats and the harm are clear, as are the needed interventions, preventative measures, and solutions. We must demand and support action.

Treat digital health tools as medical equipment

Like awareness and education, another step that can be taken now to decrease the risks of digital health in home settings is to treat digital health tools more like durable medical equipment. First, biomedical equipment management is a mature field with an extensively trained network. There is no reason to reinvent proper medical equipment setup, maintenance, or service, given that these models are readily available. Specific academic and clinical training education programs already exist as does national certification for biomedical equipment technicians.[11] Recall our discussion on hospital bed fires. All medical equipment carries risks and there already is an entire industry built around mitigating those risks.

In practice this could look very similar to how other digital technologies have evolved to support consumers. Support and maintenance for consumer electronics typically involves a registration process to track and notify users of updates and vulnerabilities. Think of how this alone would have worked in the Dexcom blood glucose monitoring case, if each of the users had received a real-time update that the system was down and that they should fall back to a manual surveillance method rather than opting everyone out, up front. Furthermore, consumer electronics manufacturers necessarily meet the consumer where they are with a strong digital presence. This includes helpful videos on YouTube, monitoring social media for misinformation and clarification, maintaining a consumer-oriented website (including frequently asked questions, easy to use hardware/software identification tool, software/firmware updates, real-time chat, and more). Integrated into this digital presence is an operations center that monitors the health of the devices and systems themselves and aggressively tracks threat and vulnerabilities through highly regarded and commercially available services. All of these factors better situates these companies to understand the health of their product lines, the satisfaction and safety of their customers, and to identify and mitigate threats proactively.

Lastly, the rapid changes in medical practice brought on by COVID-19 have proven the utility of telehealth but have also reminded us of the importance of home healthcare. If not for visiting nurses and phlebotomists, the impact on health care and clinical trials would have been far worse. Medical equipment dispensed and managed by home healthcare companies have enabled patients to continue with therapies and monitoring with less overall exposure to clinical centers for decades. Home health care organizations are expert in the training and deployment of complex medical equipment into home settings and provide sound options for digital tool delivery if they can behave like consumer electronics companies (Geek-Squad for digital health).

Professionalism and workforce development

We already touched upon the possibility of utilizing preexisting educational and certification, such as the Biomedical Engineering Technician (BMET certification) programs for digital health workforce development. This would provide a solid basis but would comprise only a single layer of the necessary workforce transformation. Clinicians in training are learning more and more about algorithms and clinical decision support tools but mostly in elective fashion. Quantitative and computer methodologies, as well as digital health tools, must become a standardized part of clinical and allied health training, especially the risk management elements.

Further, the academic, private, and public biomedical research industries must organize digital health programs around the critical competencies and experience to drive quality and safe outcomes. Cross-trained and multidisciplinary teams are essential, but so is fundamental competence. The authors have seen far too many instances of an IT professional trying to select a wearable for a clinical use case, or of a senior clinician, trying to sound authoritative on healthcare cybersecurity to be comfortable with the status quo. As more rational, formal, objective, and focused career paths emerge, quality outcomes for all parties will increase.

This simple step of including digital technologies as part of Continuing Professional Education (CPE) for medical certifications would create better awareness and understanding. There is already extensive and necessary certification for HIPAA and ELHR systems required for clinicians and researchers. Routine training around the novel risks that the use of digital health poses, perhaps using examples such as the 10 Toxicities would better serve medical personnel to understand the risks up front and recognize manifestations more quickly when they occur.

This is not meant to discount these unique career paths, quite the contrary, but it is a call for professionalism. In addition to formal training, there is also a role for professional societies in workforce professionalism. New organizations, such as the Digital Medicine Society (DiME) are leading the way but there is analogous opportunity for traditional professional societies to play a part via continued education and subspecialty creation.[12] Lastly, we should recognize and exploit our youngest emerging leaders as often having a sixth sense about technologies that many of we established professionals lack. I believe my daughter was only in middle school the first time I saw her place a piece of tape over the camera on our new TV. She then explained the risks to me . . . Just as digital health has stretched traditional medical, technological, and regulatory boundaries, it has created the demand for a specialized work-force and this opportunity is too good to pass up.

Lock and load

Clearly, the presence of an adversary is likely the most foreign element of digital health risk to medicine. Traditionally, disease and ignorance have been the main foes of medicine and science. Today, medicine is seen as fertile ground for theft, ransom, and sowing fear and chaos, and as a vector for this, medicine must find a way to respond. Using state-sponsored medical misinformation campaigns as an example, is the AMA ready to take on the KGB? Of course not, but it needs to consider this kind of threat and how this will require new partnerships among medicine, consumer regulators, the intelligence community, and federal agencies that have national defense missions. Similarly, individual clinicians who utilize social media to network and communicate must be prepared for trolls and targeted attacks, not only on their views but on them personally. In short, we must recognize that cyberspace is a wonderful but, also, a very dangerous place and that each new opportunity brings corresponding risk. As has always been the case in medicine, an ounce of prevention will always be superior to a pound of cure.

References

1. Perakslis ED. Cybersecurity in Health Care. *New England Journal of Medicine* 2014. 371(5):395–397.
2. Privacyrights.org. Data Breach Database. Downloaded January 2020. https://privacyrights.org/data-breaches
3. U.S. FDA. Cybersecurity Safety Communications. 2020, January 23. Accessed January 2020. https://www.fda.gov/medical-devices/digital-health/cybersecurity#safety
4. Davis J. When Medical Devices Get Hacked, Hospitals Often Don't Know It. *Health IT News*. 2018, May 11.
5. Bernabe RD, GJ van Thiel, JA Raaijmakers, and JJ van Delden. The Risk-Benefit Task of Research Ethics Committees: An Evaluation of Current Approaches and the Need to Incorporate Decision Studies Methods. *BMC Medical Ethics* 2012. 13:6. doi:10.1186/1472-6939-13-6
6. Juhaeri J. Benefit-Risk Evaluation: The Past, Present and Future. *Therapeutic Advances in Drug Safety* 2019. 10:2042098619871180.
7. U.S. HHS. Medical Devices; Exemption from Premarket Notification for Class I and Class II Devices. Federal Register. 2019, December 30.
8. U.S. FDA. Proposed Regulatory Framework for Modifications to AI/ML-based Software as a Medical Device (SaMD). Accessed January 2020. https://www.fda.gov/media/122535/download

9. Erwig M. Let's Stop Treating Algorithms Like They Are All Created Equal. MIT Press Reader. Accessed January 2020. https://thereader.mitpress.mit.edu/lets-stop-treating-algorithms-like-theyre-all-created-equal/

10. U.S. FDA. What are "Biologics" Questions and Answers. 2018, February 6. Accessed January 202. https://www.fda.gov/about-fda/center-biologics-evaluation-and-research-cber/what-are-biologics-questions-and-answers

11. Biomedical Equipment Certification. Accessed July 2020. https://www.healthcarepathway.com/certification/biomedical-equipment-technician-certification/

12. DiME Society Homepage. Accessed July 2020. https://www.dimesociety.org/

Index